TOTAL HEALTH
AT THE COMPUTER

TOTAL HEALTH AT THE COMPUTER

HOW TO BE PAIN FREE
& RELIEVE THE SYMPTOMS OF COMPUTER STRESS SYNDROME

MARTIN SUSSMAN & DR. ERNEST LOEWENSTEIN
with HOWARD SANN

Station Hill

Published by Station Hill Press, Barrytown, New York 12507.
Cover and book design by Susan Quasha.

Distributed by the Talman Company, 131 Spring Street, Suite 201E-N, New York, New York 10012.

Library of Congress Cataloging-in-Publication Data

Total health at the computer: a how-to guide to saving your eyes and body at the VDT screen in 3 minutes a day   /   by Martin A. Sussman... [et al.].
          p.   cn.
Includes index.
ISBN 0-88268-162-1 : $13.95
1. Video display terminals—Health aspects. 1. Sussman, Martin A., 1951-
RC965.V53T68 1991
613.6'2—dc20   93-1721
                                                    CP

Manufactured in the United States of America.

CONTENTS

DISCLAIMER

This book does not diagnose, prognose or treat any medical conditions of the eye, visual system or body. The information in this book does not and cannot take the place of regular eye and body care with a qualified, licensed practitioner. If your symptoms persist, consult a vision specialist or a medical doctor. Anyone with a medical problem or medical disorder is advised to consult an eye doctor or general physician.

ACKNOWLEDGEMENTS

To Janet Parker, for all the illustrations and diagrams that make the information in this book so much easier to grasp and understand.

To Dr. Allan H. Verter, chiropractor, for his expertise on how to sit correctly at the computer.

To Sharon Lyon, massage therapist, for her assistance in choosing the exercises for repetitive strain injury, carpal tunnel syndrome and arm, hand and shoulder problems.

FROM HEADACHES TO HEALTH

At first glance it seems that using a computer is bad for you. At least judging by the number of complaints and the severity of them — operators wearing splints and needing surgery on tendons and wrists — it certainly seems that computer work is taxing and painful.

More than 50 million people now spend at least part of each day parked in front of computer screens; perhaps 25 million of them spend *most* of their days working at video display terminals (VDTs). The numbers will continue to rise in a society increasingly focused on computer literacy. If the current trend continues, it's predicted that by 1997 more than half of the U.S. workforce will be using VDTs on a daily basis.[1]

State of the office

Computer users report a wide range of discomforts: Headaches; neck aches, shoulder tightness and back problems; and elbow, forearm, wrist, hand and finger problems.

And more: physical and mental fatigue. That familiar wiped-out feeling after work.

Add to that a new wrinkle: vision problems and problems with the eyes.

Why are millions of people — students, secretaries, data entry operators, computer programmers, telephone operators, accountants, reporters, editors, corporate executives, people from all walks of life — experiencing so much pain and discomfort from performing a task that involves only the hands and the eyes?

The problem would *seem* to be in the nature of the work itself — long hours sitting stiffly in one place staring at a computer screen.

But the fact is: *There is nothing inherent in computer work that causes pain, physical discomfort or poor vision.*

You do not have to endure pain as the price of working at a computer — in the corporate world, in school, in your office or wherever your job is.

RSI and computer work

And yet, in 1981, according to the U.S. Bureau of Labor Statistics, repetitive strain injury (RSI) — the term used to describe some of the aches and pains of what can only be called Computer Stress Syndrome — accounted for 18 percent of workplace illness (23,000 out of a reported 126,000 cases of occupational illness). By 1987, the number of cases of RSI had tripled (72,900) and, by 1989, repetitive strain injuries were accounting for 50 percent of all job illnesses (146,900 out of 283,700). In 1990 alone, over 125,000 workers' compensation claims for carpal tunnel syndrome were submitted[2] ; double the number filed in 1988.[3] RSI at its worst, carpal tunnel syndrome can cause numbness, pain or tingling sensations in the thumb and fingers. It's been estimated that one case of carpal tunnel syndrome can cost an employer between $30,000 and $100,000. Repetitive strain injuries remain the leading workplace illness with 223,600 cases reported in 1991.

In October of 1992 — in its most comprehensive look at the relationship between work on VDTs and RSI to date — the National Institute of Occupational Safety and Health (NIOSH) revealed the results of a two-year study of 1,000 *Los Angeles Times* employees. One finding: The more hours a day a worker spends on a VDT, the greater the odds that he or she will develop hand or wrist injuries.

Dr. Bruce Bernard, a NIOSH medical officer who supervised the study, said this link, while seemingly obvious, is not widely recognized. He raised the possibility that employers might need to redesign workplaces. *The Los Angeles Times* is already doing this.[4]

It comes as no surprise that *The New York Times* referred to computer offices as "electronic sweat shops of the 90s."

The toll on the eyes

Visual ailments and visual symptoms have become major problems as well.

People who have never needed glasses sit down to work at a computer and before long they've got their first prescriptions. And people who have been using glasses sit down at a computer monitor and find themselves needing stronger and stronger prescriptions over shorter and shorter periods of time.

Eyestrain, in fact, *is* the most common complaint of computer users.

The American Optometric Association says that 50 to 75 percent of all VDT workers report eye problems.[5] The journal, *Survey of Ophthalmology*, said the numbers were even greater — with between 45 and 94 percent of computer users complaining of visual problems. And, in still another survey conducted by SteelCase, Inc., eyestrain again was the most-often reported problem.

According to a 1991 survey of optometrists, 8 million people are showing up each year at their eye doctors complaining of VDT-related problems.[6]

How we got here

This wasn't the case in the office when people worked at typewriters. Typing-related injuries were not at epidemic level and a large percentage of the workforce wasn't reeling from repetitive strain injuries.

What happened?

Overtly, there were two major changes. With the advent of computers, the page — which was paper, on a horizontal surface and could be moved to a comfortable position — became a polished glass screen, inverted to a fixed vertical position with limited adjustability for comfort.

At least, these were the most obvious changes.

Concurrently, there was no change in office furniture. Offices weren't designed or built for computer use. Neither was lighting.

When computers came in, the desks that typewriters sat on simply became computer desks. And the fixed relationship between the keyboard and the screen required workers to hold a relatively immobile posture for a long time. Advances in internal communications (i.e., computer mailboxes) further eliminated alternate tasks that up until then had allowed operators (and before them typists) to leave their desks and move around the office. So operators wound up sitting in front of their workstations even longer.

The concept of ergonomics — the science that coordinates office design with workers' needs — had taken a backseat to performance.

The phenomenon of glare

Along with computers came glare, a new phenomenon that posed greater and more serious problems, and the only available solutions were ones that created postural distortions — operators having to tilt, twist and angle their bodies to get away from annoying and irritating reflections.

Back then there was no history, experience or understanding of the fatiguing impact of glare — physically, mentally or visually — much less any guidelines to eliminate it.

Office work *might* have been streamlined into a new technology, but the workers certainly hadn't been. The workers were only taught how to operate the computers and use the software.

No one was ever taught how to correctly use his or her body, eyes and mind during computer work. And no one was ever taught what he or she *really* needed to know to take care of him or herself and be healthy, relaxed and productive at the computer.

The problem and the solution

One reason that you were probably never taught what you needed to know to be healthy at the computer was that most people have been too busy blaming the computer instead of training the operator.

Another reason is that no one ever made the connection between certain symptoms and what really causes them.

For example, blurred or double vision and slow refocusing are generally recognized as vision problems. But a host of other problems — such as losing one's place while inputting data, skipping words or lines, losing comprehension or attention, and difficulty maintaining concentration — long considered performance problems are actually vision problems in disguise.

The good news is that certain vision problems *are* correctable *and can be* reversed. Many people do not know this.

Also, while many people understand the importance of exercise and training to keep the body in shape, many people are equally *un*aware that exercise and training techniques *also exist for the eyes* — to reduce and eliminate current vision problems and prevent future ones.

There *is* a direct relationship between your body, your vision and your performance. Stress on the body creates stress on the visual system which creates stress on the body, which in turn creates stress on performance (i.e., less effective and less productive).

But it *is* possible to work at a computer with considerably less effort and less fatigue.

How? — By learning how to correctly use your eyes, your body and your mind at the computer.

This is the way that you can reduce and eliminate long-term eyestrain, nagging headaches and other vision- or body-related problems.

It *is* possible to work at a computer for long hours, be healthy and even feel energized. It *can* be done.

This book will show you how.

What this book will show you

This book will teach you how to feel good after a day at the computer.

It will tell you what to do and show you how to do it. You will find it easy to work with and incorporate into your daily routine.

There are some very simple but effective adjustments that you can make in your workspace that will help you eliminate stress. How to solve the problem of glare, for one.

And, with a few minor changes in how you sit at the computer and how you position yourself in relation to the VDT screen and your keyboard, you can eliminate many, if not all, of the external causes of both physical and mental tension and fatigue.

Also, by learning how to properly use your eyes and how to rest your eyes, you will be able to reduce or eliminate most eye problems and nagging headaches.

This book will directly address the five factors that cause the aches, pains and discomforts that are symptoms of Computer Stress Syndrome.

You will learn how to:
- Properly set up (or better adjust) your computer workspace
- Correctly use your body at the computer
- Correctly use your eyes at the computer
- Correctly choose the appropriate glasses for computer work
- Eliminate accumulated stress and strain
- Attain optimum visual fitness and performance

By applying the principles in this book you can develop healthy techniques at the computer and eliminate the pains that have been plaguing you.

You will also learn how to enhance your physical comfort and well being, sharpen your mental alertness, and maintain visual clarity with much greater ease.

[1] James LaRue, "Terminal Illnesses," *Wilson Library Bulletin,* September 1991, pp. 85-88.

[2] Bristol Voss, "Health Hazards: Hidden Perils in the Workplace," *Sales & Marketing Management*, November 1991, pp. 127-128.

[3] Diana Hembree, "Warning: Computing Can Be Hazardous To Your Health," *MacWorld*, January 1990, pp. 150-157.

[4] Bob Baker, "NIOSH Study Backs Claims of Stress Injury," *Los Angeles Times*, 29 October 1992, pp. D1, D5 and "Time at the Keyboard is an RSI risk at the *LA Times*," *VDT NEWS*, November/December 1992, pp. 3-4.

[5] Voss, p. 128.

[6] "State of the Office," *VDT NEWS*, January/February 1992, p. 5 (from a survey for Optical Coating Laboratory, Inc., Santa Rosa, CA).

HOW TO USE THIS BOOK

This book is your guide to health, comfort and relief from the pain of working at the computer.

In the first chapter of Part One you will be introduced to the Nine Fundamentals — habits to practice while you are at the computer.

The second chapter discusses the glasses and contacts that are best to use at the computer.

If you currently are not experiencing any pain, tension, stress or vision problems at the computer, the consistent application of the principles in these first two chapters will help you maintain your current symptom-free state.

If you are currently experiencing any of the symptoms of Computer Stress Syndrome, you will find *Chapter Three* to be your doorway to relief. All of the most common symptoms are listed alphabetically there, together with techniques for relieving them and advice for preventing their occurrence. Simply look up your symptom in the alphabetical listing and you will be led to the relevant parts of this book. These will include reference to 1. The specific "fundamentals" that apply to your symptom, and 2. The "3-minute routine" designed to relieve it. These exercises that comprise the routines are given in Chapter Four of this part of the book (Pp. 49-92).

Prolonged work at a computer places unique demands on your visual system. Part Two explains what these demands are as well as what visual skills are necessary to meet those demands. You will also be introduced to a Vision Enhancement Training that will help you improve your visual skills and maintain good vision. Practice this training regularly if you find that the visual symptoms of Computer Stress Syndrome are not helped by the 3-minute routines in Part One.

Part Three discusses the possible health risks posed by computer monitors. As well as gaining a background in this important subject, you will also learn specific steps to take to minimize your exposure to electromagnetic radiation.

The Appendix contains the eye charts needed for some of the exercises, information about behavioral optometry and a special note to employers of people who use computer technology in their business.

THE SYMPTOMS OF COMPUTER STRESS SYNDROME

Below are listed the most common symptoms of Computer Stress Syndrome (CSS) reported by computer users.

Symptoms are grouped according to the main area they affect, but most do not exist alone. Since there is a direct relationship between your vision, your body and your performance, you will probably experience more than one symptom if you experience any at all. Before proceeding it might be helpful for you to read through this list in order to locate the symptoms you need to work on.

BODY PROBLEMS
> Drowsiness, fatigue, feeling tired when rested
> Headaches after near work
> Headaches around eyes/Eyes hurt
> Headaches, front brow (forehead)
> Headaches, back, sides or top of head
> Headaches late in day
> Pain in thighs, legs, lower back
> Tingling and pain in arms, wrists, hands
> Tension in upper body (neck, back, shoulders, arms)

EYE PROBLEMS
> Excessive blinking
> Eyes hurt, ache, strain, pull, sting, burn, tear, itch
> Rubbing eyes

VISION PROBLEMS
> Blurred distance vision after computer work
> Blurred near vision/Screen goes in and out of focus
> Blurred vision as day progresses
> Double vision at screen

VISION PROBLEMS (*continued*)
    Glasses don't "feel" right/Need stronger glasses
    Headaches
    Slow refocusing ability
    Squinting to see

CONCENTRATION AND PERFORMANCE PROBLEMS
(Most often directly associated with vision problems)
    Difficulty concentrating/Short attention span
    Irritability during or after computer work
    Losing place, skipping, repeating lines
    Misaligning columns, interchanging words or numbers

Causes of Computer Stress Syndrome

The different symptoms of Computer Stress Syndrome are most often the result of five major factors:

- The incorrect use of the eyes and body during computer work
- The use of inappropriate glasses or contact lenses for computer work
- The improper set up of the computer workspace
- The accumulation of physical, mental and visual strain
- A less-than-optimal level of visual fitness necessary for the demands of computer work.

Part One

STAYING HEALTHY AND GETTING RELIEF

The Nine Fundamentals of being healthy at the computer

How to set up your computer workspace

FUNDAMENTAL 1: **Maximize Focusing Distance**
FUNDAMENTAL 2: **Eliminate Glare**
FUNDAMENTAL 3: **Light The Room Appropriately**

How to use your body at the computer

FUNDAMENTAL 4: **Position Yourself Correctly**
FUNDAMENTAL 5: **Sit and Bend Properly**
FUNDAMENTAL 6: **Breathe Regularly and Relax Your Body**

How to use your eyes at the computer

FUNDAMENTAL 7: **Blink Every 3 to 5 Seconds**
FUNDAMENTAL 8: **See More Than The Screen**
FUNDAMENTAL 9: **Look Into The Distance Frequently**

One Woman's Story

A 30-something woman finally landed the plum job she'd wanted all her life — senior editor at a major New York publishing house.

Her first day she noticed two women working at computers with splints on their arms.

"What happened to them?" she asked.

"Oh, that's from computer work," someone told her.

"That won't ever happen to me," she told herself.

Two weeks later, her arm was in a splint.

She would be on "sick leave" for six months.

After a series of therapies she wasn't any better and realized that her choices were two: go back to the job of her dreams and endure the ever-increasing pain of carpal tunnel syndrome or get another job. She quit, remains in pain, and has filed a lawsuit.

She is not alone.

HOW TO SET UP
YOUR COMPUTER WORKSPACE

The ideal computer workspace

The ideal computer workspace contains seven key components. Having all seven will afford you the opportunity for maximum comfort at the computer, keeping you productive, relaxed and efficient throughout the day. Let's look at them. They are:

- a computer desk — with an adjustable platform for the keyboard.
- an extra-long keyboard cable — to allow you to move the keyboard to your lap or any other comfortable place.
- an adjustable chair — for both the chair height *and* the chair back.
- a large-screen monitor — with adjustable brightness and contrast controls.
- an anti-glare screen — to free your VDT screen from reflected glare.
- a tilt-and-swivel stand for the monitor — to adjust the screen to the proper angle.
- an upright stand for your copy — so you don't have to look back and forth, down at the desk and up to the screen.

But it's more than likely that you work in an office or at a computer workstation that was set up long before you got there. Or that, even if you had played a role in setting up your office space, you may not have been aware of what the ideal components were. And now you might not be able to start all over again.

Don't despair. Even if you don't have any (or very few) of the ideal components, you can still achieve a significantly higher level of health and comfort at the computer by *making the changes that are available and possible for you.* In fact, you have more control than you think.

Gaining control — a logical approach

First, analyze your current situation to see *how you can make the components adjustable to you* rather than you adjusting to them. This is crucial.

For example, if you don't have a tilt-and-swivel stand for your monitor, to avoid having to tilt your head to see the screen you can readjust the height of your chair or you can put a book under the front of the monitor to tilt the screen to the proper angle. And if you don't have an adjustable chair, you can sit on a pillow or a phone book.

The point is: you don't have to endure your work environment as is. Learn the components of the ideal workspace and the Nine Fundamentals of Being Healthy at the Computer (in the next section) and then ask yourself, *"What can be adjusted to make me more comfortable?"* Only then can you begin to see the possibilities that you may have overlooked.

Again, at your office, ask yourself: *"What is the scope of the area within which I can make changes without going to my employer or overstepping my boundaries?"*

Once you assume this responsibility, you will be able to respond more effectively to make your workspace more comfortable and efficient. This, in turn, will increase your overall effectiveness and productivity.

Second, implement the adjustments that you know you can make now. This may mean having to overcome an initial resistance to change, which sounds something like this: *"I don't have time, I'm too busy and under too much pressure to stop working to rearrange furniture."*

Remember, you *are* worth the time and effort it takes to make the simple, necessary and pivotal adjustments that will make your workspace healthier for you.

In the long run, your wellbeing and your work both suffer when you are not performing at an optimum level of comfort.

Even if you have absolutely no control over your workspace and cannot make any adjustments to it, changing how you use your body and your eyes at the computer will make a major difference in your overall efficiency and effectiveness.

Make a conscious choice for better health and implement the changes. With the right attitude you can overcome almost any physical limitation that you might face and take a major step in relieving your pain and discomfort.

How to set up your workspace

In deciding where to set up your computer in your office the three fundamentals to apply are:

- **Maximize Focusing Distance** (*Fundamental 1*)
- **Eliminate Glare** (*Fundamental 2*)
- **Light The Room Appropriately** (*Fundamental 3*)

Achieving these basics will create an environment in which you can optimally *use* and *rest* your eyes. It will also give you a head start in being able to eliminate two of the major sources of physical and mental fatigue — glare and eyestrain.

FUNDAMENTAL 1

Maximize Focusing Distance

Set your computer up in your workspace so that you can look beyond the screen to the farthest object in the room.

Being able to look up into the distance is the most important way that you can rest your eyes during computer work. Rest also prevents the accumulation of visual stress.

If possible, you *don't* want to be in the corner of the room or face a wall or window. Window light is another source of unwanted stress. Instead, try facing a doorway so your distance view is down the hall.

FUNDAMENTAL 2

Eliminate Glare

Glare is any light or image reflected off the VDT screen that reaches the eyes, cannot be ignored and competes for visual attention.

Sources of glare may be the lights in the room, the light fixtures themselves, unshaded windows, or bright objects, such as your own white shirt or blouse.

Glare silently forces you to (unconsciously) twist and turn your head and body to avoid it. And your eyes *do* have to work harder to focus on the information on the screen (which leads to eyestrain and strains of the neck, back, shoulders and arms).

You can tell there's reflected glare by turning on the lights in the room before turning on your computer. If you see any images or reflections on the (turned-off) screen, you've got a glare problem.

To reduce or minimize glare, experiment by:
- Tilting the screen
- Moving objects that reflect *onto* the screen
- Covering windows to block sunlight
- Turning off or lowering offending lights
- Covering fluorescent lights with egg-crate baffles
- Turning your computer so the screen is perpendicular to overhead fluorescent lights.

This may do it. However, since most offices were not designed or built for computer work it may be impossible to eliminate glare altogether.

Another form of glare is light that originates from the computer screen itself. This happens when the brightness control is turned up too high and you are viewing dark letters against a bright background.

Anti-glare screens

If the lighting in your workspace is good, you will not need a glare screen.

If it isn't, adding an anti-glare screen to your monitor is a way to filter out unwanted glare, and a wise investment in your health and comfort. A good anti-glare screen increases the contrast of characters against the background, making it easier for your eyes to see.

Low-quality screens should be avoided because they can cut down the resolution and clarity of the characters on the screen, which encourages eyestrain and fatigue.

Anti-glare sprays are also available, but anti-glare screens are more effective.

Tinted glasses

Many offices are over illuminated and often overhead lights cannot be turned off. If your workstation is well laid out and you have good control of ambient lighting, most of the time a tint on your glasses won't be necessary. But if you cannot control ambient lighting it is worth discussing with an optometrist whether or not you should use tinted glasses.

For an amber screen, a light-blue or blue-gray tint is recommended. For a green screen, a rose or light-pink tint. In some cases a coating to block ultraviolet light provides increased comfort; in others, a light-gray or brown tint helps reduce the effects of excessive illumination.

FUNDAMENTAL 3

Light The Room Appropriately

If you've completely eliminated all sources of glare onto your screen, chances are your workspace is now pretty dark. This is a problem because you don't want to be working in a darkened room.

Make sure that you have some overhead, background or foreground lighting.

And make sure you don't have a light source anywhere in your line of sight when you're looking at the screen. This will distract your peripheral vision and cause mental fatigue.

Light your original copy

You also need to light any original copy that you are working from. A desk lamp with an adjustable neck works well. Just make sure that this light doesn't distract you or spill onto your VDT screen.

If you have some control over the overhead illumination, adjustable incandescent light, especially indirect light, is often the most comfortable. Standing lamps that direct light at the ceiling provide the best indirect light. If there is no dimmer available, a 3-way fixture is recommended so you can set the light at the most comfortable level .

Fluorescent Light Tip

Do fluorescent lights bother your eyes or reflect onto your screen? Most problems are caused by the *quantity* of the light (not by fluorescence itself). If possible, turn off every other fluorescent fixture and light your desk with a 100-watt bulb. Or replace all fluorescent lights with Vita-Lite®, a special fluorescent tube which emits a different *quality* of light that simulates the full spectrum of natural sunlight more closely than any other artificial light. This makes it easier on your eyes to see. (Reduce the quantity of light even if you use Vita-Lite®.)

One Young Man's Story

A 20-something man with good vision (he'd never worn glasses) worked part time at a jewelry store doing engravings. After work he played rightfield on a softball team. A solid defensive player, he was known for always getting a good jump on the ball. That is, until he got a full-time job at an accounting firm and started working at a portable computer.

At the end of his second week working at the computer he went to play softball. Suddenly, at the crack of the bat, he didn't know which way to move — whether to come in or go back. Balls started dropping in front of him and sailing over his head. And, even more suddenly, he "couldn't see any more."

After one month at the computer, his eyes hurt, he went to an eye doctor, and before the softball season ended was wearing his first pair of glasses.

HOW TO USE YOUR BODY AT THE COMPUTER

To use your body effectively while doing computer work, the three fundamentals to apply are:

- **Position Yourself Correctly** (*Fundamental 4*)
- **Sit and Bend Properly** (*Fundamental 5*)
- **Breathe Regularly and Relax Your Body** (*Fundamental 6*)

Correct posture, correct positioning and proper use of your body at the computer will keep you healthy physically and prevent symptoms of Computer Stress Syndrome and repetitive strain injuries to your arms, wrists, hands and fingers.

FUNDAMENTAL 4

Position Yourself Correctly (*See Fig. 1*)

Distance from screen

Sit so that your eyes are 18 to 24 inches from the screen.

Eyes above screen

Sit at a height so that your eyes are 6 to 8 inches above the center of the screen.

Fingers level with or below wrists, wrists level with or below elbows

Your fingers move most freely when they are level with or hang slightly below your wrists. Your wrists should also be level with or slightly below your elbows and your arms low enough so you can drop and relax your shoulders. (This will help keep your arms relaxed.)

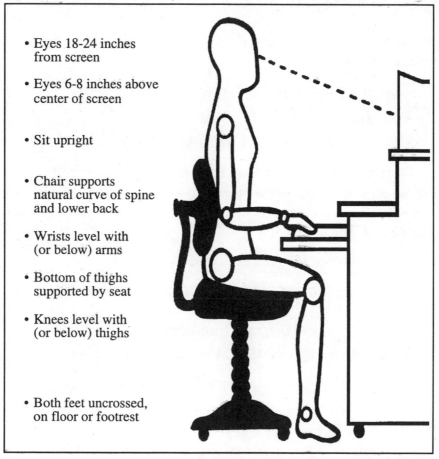

- Eyes 18-24 inches from screen

- Eyes 6-8 inches above center of screen

- Sit upright

- Chair supports natural curve of spine and lower back

- Wrists level with (or below) arms

- Bottom of thighs supported by seat

- Knees level with (or below) thighs

- Both feet uncrossed, on floor or footrest

FIG. 1 How to position yourself in relation to your computer workstation.

Bending your hands upwards as you type tightens your wrists and forearm muscles and leads to physical stress and tension *(Fig. 1)*. It can also lead to carpal tunnel syndrome — pressure on the main nerve of the wrist — which causes debilitating pain and numbness, and even permanent nerve damage if not caught and corrected in time.

The main causes of repetitive strain injuries are incorrect posture, incorrect positioning, and the improper relationships between the hands, wrists and elbows. This is why it is so important to be able to adjust the height and angle of the keyboard and the height of your chair and your chair back.

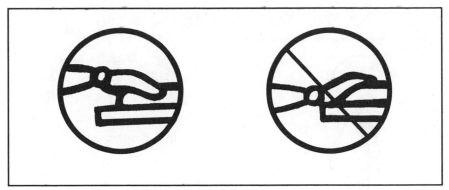

FIG. 2 Hands level with or slightly below your arms.

FUNDAMENTAL 5

Sit and Bend Properly

The key to positioning yourself correctly in front of your computer screen is to sit correctly and to pay attention to the angle of the hinge points of your body *(Fig. 1)*.

The basics of correct seated posture:

Keep your spine straight

Sit upright, keeping your spine straight.

Keep your head upright and straight too—not craned forward or dropped, not tilted or turned, and not favoring one eye over the other.

Avoid the common tendency to slouch.

Sitting upright allows you to breathe fully, regularly and easily (with no pressure on your lungs, upper chest or diaphragm).

Good posture also maximizes the flow of oxygen to all parts of your body.

Support your lower back

Sit all the way back in your chair so that your thighs are supported by the seat and your buttocks touch the chair back. If you must sit forward then put a pillow or cushion between you and the back of the chair. If you are sitting on a wedge cushion, it is not necessary that your back touch the chair back.

Make Your Chair Adjust to You

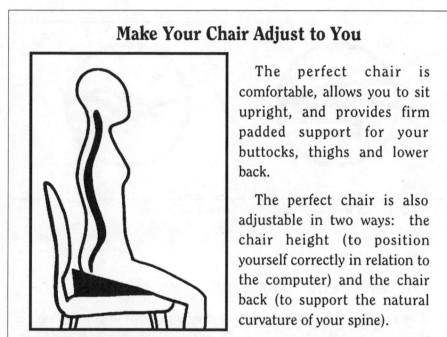

The perfect chair is comfortable, allows you to sit upright, and provides firm padded support for your buttocks, thighs and lower back.

The perfect chair is also adjustable in two ways: the chair height (to position yourself correctly in relation to the computer) and the chair back (to support the natural curvature of your spine).

Fig. 3 Using a wedge cushion.

If you cannot buy a new chair, consider using a wedged seat cushion (See illustration). This helps eliminate much of the stress that sitting places on your body by shifting the center of gravity of your body forward, thereby relieving pressure on your lower back. (Alternatively — although not as beneficial as a wedged cushion — you could sit on a phonebook to bring you up to the right height or sit on a pillow to soften the seat.)

Knees level with or below thighs

Raise the height of your chair (or use a cushion) so that your knees are level with or slightly below your thighs. This will create the proper foundation for correct seated posture and help eliminate any nagging leg tension.

Both feet on the floor, legs uncrossed

Keeping both feet on the floor provides a solid foundation for relaxed posture and helps prevent unwanted tensions and imbalances in the body. Keeping your legs uncrossed facilitates better circulation.

If your feet don't touch the floor, use a phone book or foot rest.

Body maintains itself upright without arm support

Your body, from the waist up, should maintain itself in an upright position (again, without slouching or sagging). Do not use your arms to hold your trunk or body upright.

Your arms may rest on the desk or chair arms, but if they do, make sure you don't slouch your back or shift your weight. Keep your weight in the center of your seat.

Bend from the waist

When you have to bend or lean forward do so from the waist, again making sure not to slouch or sag.

Bending from the mid-back cuts off the oxygen supply to the brain and strains the low back and neck, causing physical and mental fatigue.

Bending correctly from the waist keeps your energy flowing and strengthens the musculature that supports your spinal column.

Sit Tip

The most common habit of improper posture when sitting is for the lower back (lumbar region) to curve backward in a slouch rather than slightly forward. Instead, sit upright, keeping your spine straight *(Fig. 4A)*. Avoid letting your pelvis slide forward (slouching) or dropping (sagging) your mid-back against the chair back *(Fig. 4B)*.

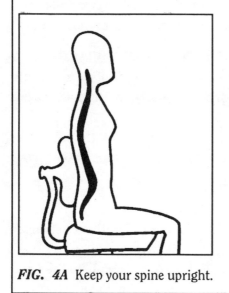

FIG. 4A Keep your spine upright.

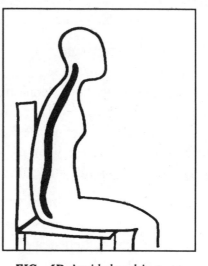

FIG. 4B Avoid slouching.

FUNDAMENTAL 6

Breathe Regularly and Relax Your Body

Breathe regularly and easily

Deep breathing and proper relaxation will make it easier for you to concentrate at the computer for longer periods of time.

Breathing too shallowly, irregularly or holding your breath creates tension, stress and fatigue. Holding your breath is a sign of "tense" mental concentration, which is taxing on your mind and draining on your body.

You might have already noticed that most times when you are in a pressure situation, feel tense or are in a bad mood, the rhythm and pace of your breathing changes. Remember to keep breathing. As simple as it seems, it helps keep you relaxed and mentally alert.

(See Deep Breathing exercise on P. 62.)

Keeping your body relaxed

When sitting, keep your body relaxed and pay particular attention to relaxing your forehead (brow), neck, back and jaw.

As we mentioned before, relax your shoulders and let your arms fall relaxed at your sides with your elbows bent comfortably.

Relax Tip

When you become aware of tension in a part of your body while working, here is a quick and easy way to relax your body: Take a deep breath and tense that part (as tight as you can!) as you hold the inhale for 3 to 5 seconds. Relax as you exhale. Repeat if necessary.

One Man's Story

A 40-something man who had worn glasses for 32 years (nearsighted with a severe astigmatism) got a job in word processing. Over the next three years he spent a minimum of 8 hours a day working at a computer. His eyesight improved!

How?

During the second year, he took a vision seminar to see if there was anything he could do to improve his eyesight. There was.

The seminar led him to a behavioral optometrist who directed him through vision therapy for four months, a half-hour a week.

After a weekend with a migraine headache, he reported to his weekly session and — for the first time in over 3 decades — was able to read the 20/20 line on the eye chart with his astigmatic eye and without glasses.

"You don't need glasses anymore," his optometrist told him. "Go to the Registry of Motor Vehicles and get the restriction off your license."

He did it and hasn't worn glasses since.

HOW TO USE YOUR EYES AT THE COMPUTER

To keep your vision as clear and relaxed as it can be, these are the three fundamentals you want to practice, integrate and use while working at the computer:

- **Blink Every 3 to 5 Seconds** *(Fundamental 7)*
- **See More Than The Screen** *(Fundamental 8)*
- **Look Into The Distance Frequently** *(Fundamental 9)*

Correct blinking, "opening up" your vision (being aware of your surroundings while looking at the screen), and taking short vision breaks will keep your eyes healthy and relaxed, your vision clear, and increase your ability and ease to concentrate.

FUNDAMENTAL 7

Blink Every 3 to 5 Seconds

Blinking lubricates and cleanses the eyes, keeping them moist for clear vision and comfort. Blinking also helps relax the facial muscles and forehead, countering the tendency to furl one's brow and create tension.

Many people do not blink regularly. Instead, while concentrating under pressure, they keep their eyes wide open — fixed — and blinking decreases. Decreased blinking often causes redness, burning and itching of the eyes, particularly for those who use contact lenses.

How to Blink Correctly:

- Move only your eyelids — not your forehead, face or cheeks.
- Make sure you close your eyes all the way without effort and that both the upper and lower lids touch gently.
- Make sure that your brow is relaxed.
- Blink lightly every 3 to 5 seconds.

(See Blinking Exercises on Pp. 53 and 71.)

FUNDAMENTAL 8

See More Than The Screen

Keep your vision "open."

This means that while looking at the screen you are also aware of your surroundings — the desk, the walls, people passing by, etc. Using your peripheral vision can significantly reduce visual stress, physical fatigue and mental tiredness.

You can expand your peripheral vision when looking directly at something by reminding yourself to be aware of objects to your right and left.

Total visual awareness promotes visual, physical and mental relaxation and will help you see more easily and clearly.

FUNDAMENTAL 9

Look Into The Distance Frequently

Extended staring at a computer screen inevitably creates fatigue, tension and eye problems. Failing to take short vision breaks is one of the major factors leading to nearsightedness among computer users. Don't wait for your eyes to start hurting or for your vision to get blurry before taking short vision breaks on a regular basis.

Simple as it seems, a brief look into the distance every 2 to 3 minutes prevents the build-up of visual stress and discomfort and keeps your eyes healthy and active.

And, contrary to conventional wisdom, a break every hour — however long it might be — does not provide all the relief and rest that your eyes need. But a short vision break is effective and beneficial. Actually, this short break takes less time than a 5-minute break every hour.

Taking short vision breaks doesn't require "real" time, only "real" awareness, an awareness that you can develop.

Short vision breaks will keep your eye muscles relaxed and flexible and prevent the accumulation of visual stress and fatigue. They'll also increase your ability to maintain concentration for longer periods of time as well as increase your accuracy and productivity over that period of time.

Hard copy — where to put it?

Ideally, you want your copy on the same plane as the screen — vertical. Working side to side is preferable to looking from the screen down to your copy and then back up to the screen again, ad infinitum.

Alternate moving the written material that you work from to the left and right of the screen during the day. The eye movements required to shift back and forth from left to right and from screen to copy — help reduce visual stress. This will enhance your visual skills.

Short Vision Break Tip

- Look up and focus on the furthest object in the distance.
- Be aware of objects around you in your periphery.
- Take a deep breath. Relax on the exhale.
- Blink correctly a couple of times.
- Shift your vision back to the screen and refocus.
  (Three near-to-far shifts per break are recommended.)

Peripheral Vision Tip

A thin line separates "concentration with attention" from "concentration with tension." To prevent yourself from crossing over this line keep your breathing full and relaxed, blink regularly and lightly, and "open" your peripheral vision.

Using your total visual awareness will help you focus more easily on what you are doing (concentration with attention) while at the same time prevent you from expending too much mental effort (concentration with tension).

In short, good peripheral vision helps relax your eyes and your mind.

2

WHICH GLASSES TO USE AT THE COMPUTER

All eyeglasses and contact lenses are not the same.

Whether or not you currently use either, you could benefit from using special "computer glasses." These "computer glasses" help relieve visual strain and halt the deterioration of vision that can sometimes accompany using a computer.

In fact, even if you do not presently need regular glasses or contacts, you can benefit from using "computer glasses" because they can help you maintain the good vision you already have.

In addition to using "computer glasses", applying the principles in this book will help improve your ability to function more efficiently and effectively at the computer. If you presently need glasses/contacts, the correct and consistent application of these principles can initially lead a reduction in the strength of your prescription and eventually to a reduced need to use them.

What kind of special "computer glasses" you need depends on your particular vision problem.

If you use glasses/contacts for distance vision

Most people who use glasses for distance seeing are nearsighted and without their glasses near objects are clearer than distant ones. In fact, many nearsighted people see reasonably well close-up without glasses altogether.

However, when distance glasses are used for extended near work the result is often stress, fatigue, tension and reduced performance. Why? Because your eyes have to work even harder to bring the screen (a near object) into focus. Over time, this leads to poorer vision and the need for stronger distance glasses.

What you can do

Properly prescribed "computer glasses" for near seeing can provide relief from the stress of extended close work.

"Computer glasses" reduce stress on the focusing muscles of the eyes by making screen characters appear a little larger and a little farther away.

If you use glasses/contacts for near vision

If you already have glasses for close work it does not necessarily mean that these are the ones you should be using for computer work. Near vision glasses are usually prescribed for about 16 inches viewing distance, but this may or may not be best for your particular computer situation.

If you are using bifocals you may find that the reading portion of the glasses is too low for the greatest ease of screen viewing. Your bifocals may also require you to make slight but uncomfortable adjustments of your neck (or back) to see the screen, this only adds to physical stress and discomfort by creating physical and mental fatigue.

What you can do

It is often best to have a different prescription *or* a different type of lens for your computer work.

A single-vision glass set for computer distance, or a special bifocal, trifocal or "no-line bifocal" also may be appropriate.

If you do not use any glasses/contacts

If you are reading this book and do not use glasses or contacts it is still possible that you are experiencing some kind of visual or physical problem at the computer that led you to this book.

What you can do

Even though you do not need regular everyday glasses, "computer glasses" might enhance your performance and/or help you maintain the good distance vision that you already have.

This is definitely worth looking into if you are experiencing any visual or physical problems during computer work.

3

RELIEF FOR THE SYMPTOMS OF COMPUTER STRESS SYNDROME

The Symptom List in the next section is an alphabetical listing of the most commonly reported symptoms of Computer Stress Syndrome. Under each symptom in the table you will find two things:

1. The fundamentals that relate most directly to that complaint. *(These are the fundamentals that you need to learn, practice and use.)*

2. The 3-minute routine that will relieve it. (The exercises that comprise each 3-minute routine are listed under each symptom. The instructions for the individual exercises are in *Chapter Four* of this part of the book (Pp. 49-92). *(When you first start a routine, you may find that it requires more than 3 minutes. Once you learn and become more familiar with the routines, they will take 3 minutes or less.)*

Here are the steps to take to get relief from those symptoms that are plaguing you:

Master the Nine Fundamentals

First, make sure that you are applying *all* nine fundamentals, but pay particular attention to the ones listed under your specific symptom(s) in the Symptom List. If you haven't read through all of these yet, you should do so, in order to become familiar with them. They are in *Chapter One* of this part of the book (Pp. 11-32).

It might be that you are inadvertently overlooking the one (or two) fundamental(s) of primary importance.

Until the fundamentals become second nature, you will need to continuously and consciously remind yourself how to correctly use your eyes, mind, and body in an integrated fashion at the computer.

If your body has been very tense and your posture poor at the computer, it might require patience to develop and maintain proper posture at the computer. Why? Because your body is readjusting to a new way of being and, at first, you might feel discomfort sitting correctly. In fact, initially it might feel "more comfortable" to continue to slouch than it feels to sit properly.

Use the appropriate glasses

Second, if you use glasses or lenses, make sure that the prescription you are using is the most appropriate one for the type of computer work that you do. (See *Chapter Two*, Which Glasses To Use.)

Learn, practice and master the 3-minute routines

Third, practice the 3-minute routines listed under your specific symptoms. The routines can be practiced as many times a day as you feel necessary. Each routine consists of a series of short exercises that are done in sequence. The instructions for these exercises follow the Symptom List. (Be sure to study the "General Guidelines for all Exercises" on Pp. 49-50 before doing any of the exercises.)

You may find immediate benefit from using them, but in most cases these routines take time — two or three weeks or even longer — before you start to feel their effect. In fact, at first, after doing these routines your eyes and/or body might feel more tired.

If you regularly tend to suffer from specific problems, *use the routines early in the day before the problems appear.*

If you suffer from more than one discomfort, you'll find the most benefit by practicing *all* the routines (either separately or together).

If your symptoms persist...

If these steps don't alleviate all of your symptoms and discomforts it may be that your visual system is not operating at its maximum level of fitness or that your body is carrying accumulated tension and stress.

If your eyes or vision continue to suffer, practice the Vision Enhancement Training described in Part Two: Enhancing Your Vision.

If your body still experiences discomfort, then it may be appropriate to incorporate exercise and relaxation into your routine.

SYMPTOM LIST (in alphabetical order)

SYMPTOM:
Blurred distance vision after computer work

FUNDAMENTALS TO MASTER:

Maximize Focusing Distance	15
Breathe Regularly and Relax Your Body	26
Blink Every 3 to 5 Seconds	29
Look Into The Distance Frequently	30

3-MINUTE ROUTINE:

Head Rolls	77
Near to Far Shifting: 1 Eye	80
Corner to Corner Shifting	64
Palming	86

SYMPTOM:
Blurred near vision/Screen goes in and out of focus

FUNDAMENTALS TO MASTER:

Maximize Focusing Distance	15
Breathe Regularly and Relax Your Body	26
Look Into The Distance Frequently	30

3-MINUTE ROUTINE:

Head Rolls	77
Near to Far Shifting: 1 Eye	80
Near to Far Shifting: 2 Eyes	83
Palming	86

SYMPTOM:
Blurred vision as day progresses

FUNDAMENTALS TO MASTER:

Maximize Focusing Distance	15
Eliminate Glare	16
Light The Room Appropriately	17
Breathe Regularly and Relax Your Body	26
See More Than The Screen	30
Look Into The Distance Frequently	30

3-MINUTE ROUTINE:

Head Rolls	77
Near to Far Shifting: 2 Eyes	83
Corner to Corner Shifting	64
Palming	86

SYMPTOM:
Difficulty concentrating/Short attention span

FUNDAMENTALS TO MASTER:

Maximize Focusing Distance	15
Eliminate Glare	16
Light The Room Appropriately	17
Position Yourself Correctly	21
Sit and Bend Properly	23
See More Than The Screen	30
Look Into The Distance Frequently	30

3-MINUTE ROUTINE:

Eye Stretches	70
Near to Far Shifting: 1 Eye	80
Near to Far Shifting: 2 Eyes	83
Corner to Corner Recognition	66
Palming	86

(Near to Far exercises could be alternated on a daily basis
to bring the total time to 3 minutes or under.)

SYMPTOM:
Double vision at screen *

FUNDAMENTALS TO MASTER:

Maximize Focusing Distance	15
Breathe Regularly and Relax Your Body	26
Look Into The Distance Frequently	30

3-MINUTE ROUTINE:

Head Rolls	77
Near to Far Shifting: 1 Eye	80
Near to Far Shifting: 2 Eyes	83
Palming	86

* Double vision that persists into distance viewing, particularly *after* leaving work, may be a sign of a serious problem requiring prompt attention. See a behavioral optometrist to determine if you are using the correct prescription for computer work.

SYMPTOM:
Drowsiness, fatigue, feeling tired when rested

FUNDAMENTALS TO MASTER:

Maximize Focusing Distance	15
Eliminate Glare	16
Light The Room Appropriately	17
Position Yourself Correctly	21
Sit and Bend Properly	23
Breathe Regularly and Relax Your Body	26
Look Into The Distance Frequently	30

3-MINUTE ROUTINE:

Eye Stretches	70
Near to Far Shifting: 1 Eye	80
Near to Far Shifting: 2 Eyes	83
Corner to Corner Recognition	66
Palming	86

SYMPTOM:

Excessive blinking

FUNDAMENTALS TO MASTER:

Breathe Regularly and Relax Your Body	26
Blink Every 3 to 5 Seconds	29

3-MINUTE ROUTINE:

Blinking Practice	61
Flutter Blink	74
Closed Eye Movements	62
Near to Far Shifting: 1 Eye	80
Palming	86

SYMPTOM:

Eyes hurt, ache, strain, pull, sting, burn, tear, itch

FUNDAMENTALS TO MASTER:

Breathe Regularly and Relax Your Body	26
Blink Every 3 to 5 Seconds	29

Symptoms, early in day:
3-MINUTE ROUTINE:

Blinking Practice	61
Flutter Blink	74
Closed Eye Movements	62
Palming	86

Symptoms, late in day:
3-MINUTE ROUTINE:

Head Rolls	77
Near to Far Shifting: 1 Eye	80
Corner to Corner Shifting	64
Palming	86

SYMPTOM:

Glasses don't "feel" right/Need stronger glasses *

FUNDAMENTALS TO MASTER:

Maximize Focusing Distance	15
Breathe Regularly and Relax Your Body	26
Blink Every 3 to 5 Seconds	29
Look Into The Distance Frequently	30

3-MINUTE ROUTINE:

Head Rolls	77
Near to Far Shifting: 1 Eye	80
Near to Far Shifting: 2 Eyes	83
Palming	86

* IMPORTANT: Consult a behavioral optometrist to determine if you are using the correct prescription for computer work.

SYMPTOM:

Headaches after near work

FUNDAMENTALS TO MASTER:

Maximize Focusing Distance	15
Eliminate Glare	16
Light The Room Appropriately	17
Position Yourself Correctly	21
Sit and Bend Properly	23
Breathe Regularly and Relax Your Body	26
Look Into The Distance Frequently	30

3-MINUTE ROUTINE:

Head Rolls	77
Near to Far Shifting: 1 Eye	80
Corner to Corner Shifting	64
Palming	86

SYMPTOM:
Headaches, front brow (forehead) *

FUNDAMENTALS TO MASTER:

Maximize Focusing Distance	15
Eliminate Glare	16
Light The Room Appropriately	17
Breathe Regularly and Relax Your Body	26
See More Than The Screen	30
Look Into The Distance Frequently	30

3-MINUTE ROUTINE:

Head Rolls	77
Near to Far Shifting: 1 Eye	80
Near to Far Shifting: 2 Eyes	83
Palming	86

* IMPORTANT: If headaches persist, see a behavioral optometrist to determine if you are using the correct prescription for computer work.

SYMPTOM:
Headaches, back, sides or top of head

FUNDAMENTALS TO MASTER:

Maximize Focusing Distance	15
Position Yourself Correctly	21
Sit and Bend Properly	23
Breathe Regularly and Relax Your Body	26
Look Into The Distance Frequently	30

3-MINUTE ROUTINE:

Shoulder Shrugs/Rotations	87
Head Rolls	77
Occipital Point Massage	85
Temple/Eye Massage	89
Eye Squeeze	69
Near to Far Shifting: 1 Eye	80

SYMPTOM:

Headaches around eyes/Eyes hurt

FUNDAMENTALS TO MASTER:

Maximize Focusing Distance	15
Position Yourself Correctly	21
Sit and Bend Properly	23
Breathe Regularly and Relax Your Body	26
Blink Every 3 to 5 Seconds	29
See More Than The Screen	30
Look Into The Distance Frequently	30

3-MINUTE ROUTINE:

Shoulder Shrugs/Rotations	87
Head Rolls	77
Near to Far Shifting: 1 Eye	80
Thumb Rotations	91
Palming	86

SYMPTOM:

Headaches late in day

FUNDAMENTALS TO MASTER:

Maximize Focusing Distance	15
Position Yourself Correctly	21
Breathe Regularly and Relax Your Body	26
Blink Every 3 to 5 Seconds	29
See More Than The Screen	30
Look Into The Distance Frequently	30

3-MINUTE ROUTINE:

Full Body Stretch	75
Shoulder Shrugs/Rotations	87
Head Rolls	77
Near to Far Shifting: 1 Eye	80
Corner to Corner Shifting	64
Palming	86

SYMPTOM:
Irritability during or after computer work

FUNDAMENTALS TO MASTER:

Maximize Focusing Distance	15
Eliminate Glare	16
Light The Room Appropriately	17
Position Yourself Correctly	21
Sit and Bend Properly	23
Breathe Regularly and Relax Your Body	26
See More Than The Screen	30
Look Into The Distance Frequently	30

3-MINUTE ROUTINE:

Eye Stretches	70
Near to Far Shifting: 1 Eye	80
Near to Far Shifting: 2 Eyes	83
Corner to Corner Recognition	66
Palming	86

SYMPTOM:
Losing place, skipping, repeating lines

FUNDAMENTALS TO MASTER:

Maximize Focusing Distance	15
Breathe Regularly and Relax Your Body	26
See More Than The Screen	30
Look Into The Distance Frequently	30

3-MINUTE ROUTINE:

Near to Far Shifting: 2 Eyes	83
Corner to Corner Recognition	66
Thumb Rotations	91
Palming	86

SYMPTOM:

Misaligning columns, interchanging words or numbers

FUNDAMENTALS TO MASTER:

Maximize Focusing Distance	15
Breathe Regularly and Relax Your Body	26
See More Than The Screen	30
Look Into The Distance Frequently	30

3-MINUTE ROUTINE:

Corner to Corner Recognition	66
Thumb Rotations	91
Palming	86

SYMPTOM:

Pain in thighs, legs, lower back

FUNDAMENTALS TO MASTER:

Position Yourself Correctly	21
Sit and Bend Properly	23
Breathe Regularly and Relax Your Body	26

3-MINUTE ROUTINE:

Full Body Stretch	75
Back Stretch	59
Low Back Stretch	79

SYMPTOM:

Rubbing eyes

FUNDAMENTALS TO MASTER:

3-MINUTE ROUTINE:

SYMPTOM:

Slow refocusing ability *

FUNDAMENTALS TO MASTER:

3-MINUTE ROUTINE:

* IMPORTANT: See a behavioral optometrist to determine if you are using the correct prescription for computer work.

SYMPTOM:

Squinting to see *

FUNDAMENTALS TO MASTER:

Maximize Focusing Distance	15
Breathe Regularly and Relax Your Body	26
Blink Every 3 to 5 Seconds	29
See More Than The Screen	30
Look Into The Distance Frequently	30

3-MINUTE ROUTINE:

Head Rolls	77
Near to Far Shifting: 1 Eye	80
Near to Far Shifting: 2 Eyes	83
Palming	86

* IMPORTANT: Consult a behavioral optometrist to determine if you are using the correct prescription for computer work.

SYMPTOM:

Tension in upper body (neck, back, shoulders, arms)

FUNDAMENTALS TO MASTER:

Position Yourself Correctly	21
Sit and Bend Properly	23
Breathe Regularly and Relax Your Body	26
See More Than The Screen	30

3-MINUTE ROUTINE:

Full Body Stretch	75
Corner Chest Opener	63
Back Stretch	59
Shoulder Shrugs/Rotations	87
Head Rolls	77

SYMPTOM:
   Tingling and pain in arms, wrists, hands

FUNDAMENTALS TO MASTER:

3-MINUTE ROUTINE:

4

3-MINUTE ROUTINE EXERCISES

When practicing any of the eye and body exercises always remember these general guidelines:

Maintain good posture

When seated, follow Fundamental 5 on Pp. 23-26, Sit and Bend Properly. When standing, keep in mind the following:
- Place feet about shoulder width apart.
- Distribute your weight evenly on both feet.
- Distribute your weight evenly from front to back.
- Keep your knees relaxed (not locked).

Breathe regularly and easily

You'll be surprised at how often you unconsciously hold your breath. Breathe!

Blink lightly every 3 to 5 seconds

Avoid the tendency to stare or strain when doing the eye exercises. Remember to blink lightly and often.

Keep your body as relaxed as possible

Many of us have accumulated years of physical tension and postural imbalances that make it difficult at first to really know what true relaxation feels like.

Be aware of your body and relax as much as you can. Before you begin each exercise, take a moment to scan your body and relax any tense areas that you find. You'll be surprised at your ability to isolate the tension and relax it.

Make all movements slow and smooth

Make all movements in a smooth and relaxed way whether they are eye or body movements or are small or large. ***Do not force any movements. Do not strain, push yourself or rush when practicing your exercises.*** It is better to do one exercise well than two in a hurry.

Keep a relaxed mental attitude

You will derive the most benefit by staying mentally involved in the exercises. The exercises are not meant to be practiced mechanically. Go slowly and stay comfortable throughout.

BACK STRETCH

Purpose: To relax your back muscles and increase blood flow to the muscles in your back, shoulders and upper body.

POSITION	REPETITIONS	TIME
Standing	1 time	15 - 30 seconds

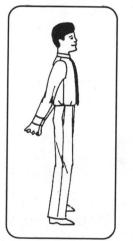

Instructions:

1. Standing with your legs shoulder-width apart and your knees relaxed and slightly bent (not locked), clasp your hands together behind your back, keeping your palms together.

2. Keeping your arms straight, slowly pull your hands and arms away from your body as far as you comfortably can. (Keep your knees slightly bent.)

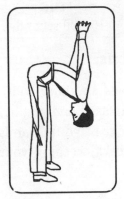

3. Now, take a deep breath and as you exhale bend over as far as you can comfortably go. Relax your head, shoulders and back. Feel the stretch in your arms and back.

Notes:

- When you clasp your hands behind your back, avoid the impulse to make your fingers touch. The correct position is for the *palms to stay together throughout the exercise*.
- You might need to learn to do this exercise in stages. For instance, it might take a while for you to be able to clasp your hands behind your back and straighten your arms. Go slow and be patient with your body.
- As always, don't force or rush any movements. Stretch only as far as comfortable and always stop before you feel resistance or strain.

BLINKING PRACTICE

Purpose: Blinking lubricates and cleanses the eyes and helps break habits of staring and "over-concentration," both of which cause visual and mental strain.

POSITION	REPETITIONS	TIME
Seated or standing	15 times	1 minute

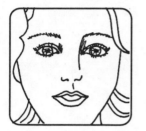

Instructions:

1. Relax your face, eyes, brow and jaw.

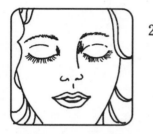

2. Close your eyes, experiencing the effortless sensation of the upper eyelids *gently* touching the lower lids. Move only your eyelids — not your forehead, face or cheeks. Relax your brow.

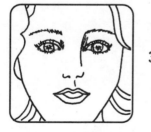

3. Open your eyes for 3 seconds.

REPEAT 14 times.

Notes:
- Do not squeeze your eyes shut when you close them. Instead, feel the lids in contact with each other without effort, without flutter and with complete relaxation of both eyes.
- Relax your eyelids when they're closed.
- Remember to breathe.

CLOSED EYE MOVEMENTS

Purpose: To relieve dry, itching or burning eyes and further lubricate and soothe the eyes.

POSITION	REPETITIONS	TIME
Seated or standing	10 times	30 - 45 seconds

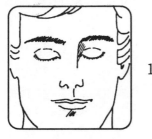

Instructions:

1. Close your eyes and keep them closed. Relax your brow.

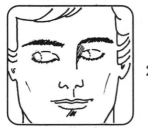

2. Slowly, move your eyes to the left and feel the stretch in the eye muscles. Hold the stretch briefly. Breathe!

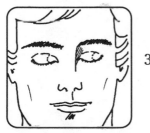

3. Now slowly move your eyes to the right and stretch. Hold the stretch briefly.

REPEAT 9 times.

Notes:

- Do not squeeze your closed eyes shut. Instead, relax the lids so that you feel no flutter.
- Do not force any stretch. Gradually, your ability to stretch your eyes further in all directions will increase.

CORNER CHEST OPENER

Purpose: To open up the upper body by stretching the pectoral, chest and shoulder muscles to free the nerve passages to the hands.

POSITION	REPETITIONS	TIME
Standing	3 times	1 1/2 minutes

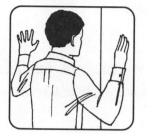

Instructions:

1. Facing a corner of a room, stand comfortably, feet shoulder-width apart and knees relaxed (slightly bent, not locked). Place your hands, palms flat, against both walls at shoulder height and exert slight pressure outward.

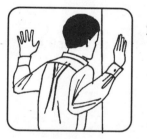

2. Now, slowly lean forward toward the corner, stopping before the point of resistance. Hold the leaned-forward position for 30 seconds. Keep your body relaxed.

REPEAT 2 times.

Notes:
- Start doing this exercise a foot and a half or more from the corner (enough distance to be able to lean forward without touching the walls). Once it is comfortable to do this exercise from this first position, take a half step (or full step) backwards and do the exercise from there.
- Feel the stretch in your pectoral muscles, chest, collarbone and shoulder blades when you are leaned forward. ***Don't bounce.***
- Breathe into the areas where you feel holding, tension or discomfort.

CORNER TO CORNER SHIFTING

Purpose: To develop central fixation — the visual skill of seeing one point best — and smoother eye movements.

POSITION	REPETITIONS	TIME
Seated	10 times (in each direction)	2 minutes

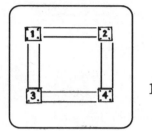

Set up:

1. Place the Computer Eye Chart (P. 143) on the four corners of your computer screen.

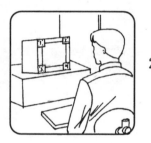

2. Sit 18 to 24 inches from your computer.

Instructions:

1. Shift your eyes from number to number using these four sequences (10 times each one).

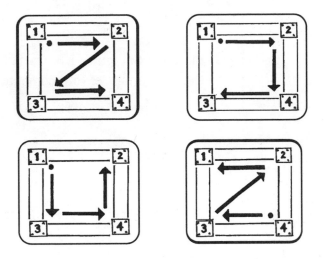

Notes:

- Adjust the speed of your shifting so that 10 rotations takes between 45 and 60 seconds.
- Remember, blink lightly and often.
- Keep your head straight and still, not tilted, turned or moving.
- Relax your forehead, jaw, neck and shoulders. If you are feeling any tension in these areas do some Head Rolls (P. 75) to relax.
- Holding your breath indicates undue effort or "trying to see." Keep breathing, regularly and easily.
- Look for the illusion of movement. When your eyes are shifting in a relaxed way, as you shift it may seem as if the chart is moving slightly in the *opposite* direction. This is what you want.

CORNER TO CORNER RECOGNITION

Purpose: To teach your mind to process visual information more easily and effectively.

POSITION	REPETITIONS	TIME
Seated	10 times (in each direction)	4 minutes

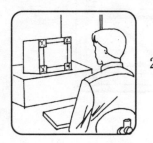

Set up:

1. Place the Computer Eye Chart (P. 143) on the four corners of your computer screen.

2. Sit 18 to 24 inches from your computer.

Instructions:

1. Shift your eyes from number to number using the following four sequences (10 times each one), calling out the number aloud as you shift to it.

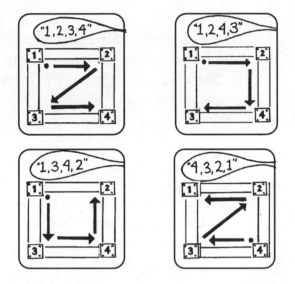

Notes:
- After you are familiar with the exercise, as you shift call out a letter in each corner instead of the number.
- Remember, blink lightly and often.
- Keep your head straight and still, not tilted, turned or moving.
- Relax your forehead, jaw, neck and shoulders. If you are feeling any tension in these areas do some Head Rolls (P. 75) to relax.
- Holding your breath indicates undue effort or "trying to see." Keep breathing, regularly and easily.
- Look for the illusion of movement. When your eyes are shifting in a relaxed way, as you shift it may seem as if the chart is moving slightly in the *opposite* direction. This is what you want.

DEEP BREATHING

Purpose: To calm the body, mind and emotions and encourage natural and relaxed breathing rhythms.

POSITION	REPETITIONS	TIME
Seated	5 times	1 - 1½ minutes

Instructions:

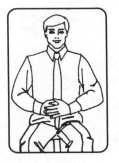

1. Sit in a comfortable position with your arms and legs uncrossed. Loosen tight clothing. Close your eyes. Place your hands on your stomach over your navel.

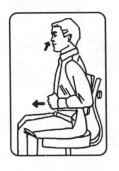

2. Inhale deeply through your nose. As you do, feel your hands rise on your belly. Hold your breath for a second or two.

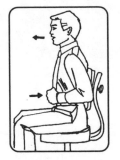

3. Now exhale gently but fully through your mouth, feeling the area under your hands collapse.

REPEAT 4 times. (Stop if you feel dizzy.)

Notes:

- When doing Deep Breathing properly, the lower abdomen and upper chest don't move, but the areas of the diaphragm just below your chest and in the lower rib cage do.
- Make sure to exhale fully and completely, expelling all the air from your lungs before you inhale again.
- Alternatively, you can do Deep Breathing while working, walking or lying down.

EYE SQUEEZE

Purpose: To increase the circulation and oxygen supply to your eyes and face, to invigorate your visual system, relax your eye muscles, break bad squinting habits and release tension.

POSITION	REPETITIONS	TIME
Seated or standing	5 times	40 seconds

Instructions:

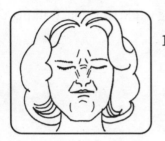

1. Inhale deeply, squeezing your eyes as tightly shut as you can. Tighten all the muscles in your neck, face and head. Tighten your jaw, too. Hold your breath for 2 to 3 seconds and continue squeezing as tightly as you can.

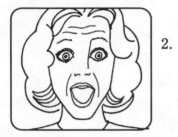

2. Now, exhale quickly, at the same time stretching your eyes wide open, opening your mouth wide, and letting out a LOUD sigh.

REPEAT 4 times.

Notes:
- Spasms or twitching in your eyelids or eye muscles is a normal response.
- Temporary flashes of clearer vision as you open your eyes is also normal.

EYE STRETCHES

Purpose: To relax and tone the six extraocular muscles surrounding your eyes.

POSITION	REPETITIONS	TIME
Seated or standing	1 time (entire set)	1 minute

Instructions:

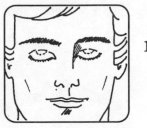

1. With your eyes closed, stretch your eyes upward, as if looking at the ceiling. Stretch and hold for 2 deep breaths then let your closed eyes return to the straight-ahead position.

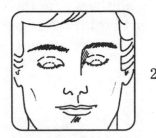

2. With your eyes still closed, stretch your eyes toward the floor. Hold this stretch for 2 deep breaths, then return your eyes straight ahead again.

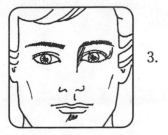

3. Open your eyes and look straight ahead. Blink lightly. Take 4 deep breaths. Relax.

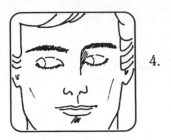

4. Close your eyes again and stretch your eyes as far to the right as you can. Stretch and hold for 2 deep breaths.

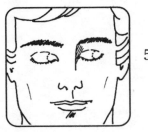

5. Now stretch your eyes all the way to the left. Again, stretch and hold for 2 deep breaths. Then return your eyes straight ahead.

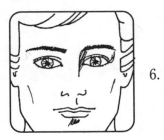

6. Open your eyes. Blink lightly. Again, take 4 deep breaths. Relax.

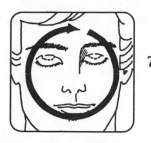

7. Close your eyes again. Now, rotate your eyes in a clockwise circle. Breathe.

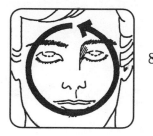

8. Lastly, rotate your eyes counter-clockwise — stretching (not straining) along the way.

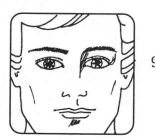

9. Now open your eyes and relax. Blink and take 4 deep breaths.

Notes:

- Make sure you keep your head still and straight and not tilted, turned or down.
- Stretch — do not strain — your eyes.
- If your eyes unconsciously "jump" out of your control or if you notice places of stiffness, tension or "stuckness," *go back over these areas slowly and gently*.
- For variety — and to work the eye muscles in different ways — you can also do Eye Stretches with your head facing in any direction: down or up, left or right, or at any angle you choose.
- With practice, your eye movements will become smoother and more fluid.

FINGER FLUTTER

Purpose: To release accumulated finger and hand tension and relax the fingers, hands and arms during computer work.

POSITION	REPETITIONS	TIME
Seated or standing	As needed	15 seconds

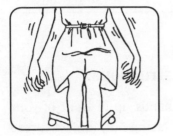

Instructions:

1. Drop your hands to your sides. Take a deep breath. On the exhale, shake your hands and fingers vigorously from the shoulders and elbows. Shake for approximately 15 seconds.

Notes:
- Relax your shoulders, arms, hands and fingers as you shake them.

FINGER STRETCH

Purpose: To stretch the muscles of the fingers, thumb and hand and to exercise the wrist; to relieve and relax the fingers, hand and forearm of tension caused by repetitive finger movements.

POSITION	REPETITIONS	TIME
Seated or standing	8 times	30 seconds

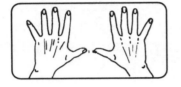

Instructions:

1. Hold both hands up in front of your face, palms facing out, fingers spread apart and your fingers and wrists fully extended and stretched.

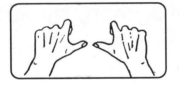

2. Starting with your little finger, quickly bend your fingers, one at a time, into a fist. Make sure that your thumbs overlap your index fingers.

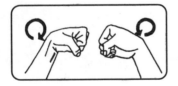

3. With your fists closed tightly, rotate your wrists 90 degrees so your fists are facing each other.

REPEAT 7 times.

Notes:
- As you make the tight fists, the idea is to close your fingers in one smooth continuous motion.
- Also, rotate *only* your wrists. Keep your elbows still as you rotate your wrists. Your forearms will rotate one quarter turn.

FLUTTER BLINK

Purpose: To reduce excessive effort while blinking, helping to relax the eyes and eye muscles.

POSITION	REPETITIONS	TIME
Seated or standing	3 sets (10 times each set)	1 minute

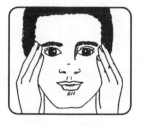

Instructions:

1. Place your fingertips gently on your temples. Blink lightly and quickly 10 times as fast as you can.

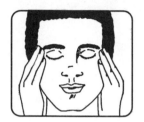

2. Now, close your eyes and rest. Take 2 or 3 deep breaths. Relax your brow and jaw.

REPEAT 2 times.

Notes:
- Make sure that with each blink you achieve full eye closure with a minimum of effort.
- You should feel *no movement* underneath your fingertips. If you feel any movement, you are blinking too hard. Use only the muscles of your eyelids (and not your facial muscles) to close your eyes.
- Remember, don't squeeze your eyes shut.

FULL BODY STRETCH

Purpose: To relax your back and shoulders and increase the body's circulation.

POSITION	REPETITIONS	TIME
Standing	3 times	30-45 seconds

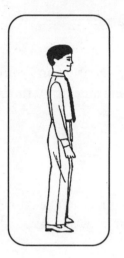

Instructions:

1. Stand with your knees relaxed (slightly bent, not locked) and your feet shoulder-width apart. Relax as you inhale.

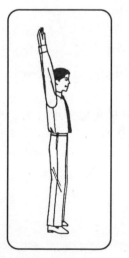

2. On the exhale, stretch both arms overhead reaching for the sky. Outstretch your fingers, arms and shoulders. Feel the stretch along both sides of your torso. Inhale.

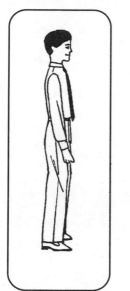

3. On the exhale, bend forward from the waist, letting your arms drop towards your toes. Relax and drop your head and neck and look toward your nose. Make sure your knees are slightly bent and not locked. Take a deep breath.

4. Now, as you exhale, slowly and gently straighten up.

REPEAT 2 times.

Notes:

- Before you start make sure you balance your weight equally on both feet and that you are equally centered fore and aft (not back on your heels or too far forward).
- Make all movements in a relaxed fluid manner, stretching — not straining — your muscles. **Don't force any movements.** Gradually your body will limber up and become more relaxed and flexible.
- Breathe deeply and slowly throughout.
- The Full Body Stretch can also be done in a sitting position.

HEAD ROLLS

Purpose: To relax your neck, head and face muscles and reduce shoulder tension.

POSITION	REPETITIONS	TIME
Standing	3 times (in each direction)	1 - 1½ minutes

Instructions:

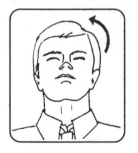

1. Take a deep breath and close your eyes. On the exhale, slowly drop your chin to your chest. Relax your neck and shoulders.

2. As you inhale deeply again, slowly and gently roll your head around to the left, then back, keeping your shoulders still and relaxed. Make your movements slowly, carefully and deliberately.

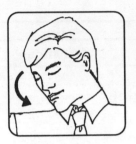

3. Now, exhale fully as you roll your head to the other side and down to your chest again.

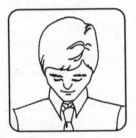

REPEAT 2 times,

then change directions and REPEAT 3 times.

Notes:
- How large a head movement you make is not as important as is moving *slowly without forcing* any movements. Be gentle.
- Again, breathe fully and deeply and relax your body.

LOW BACK STRETCH

Purpose: To relieve any pain in the legs and thighs and stretch the lower back.

POSITION	REPETITIONS	TIME
Seated	1 time (each leg)	30 seconds (each leg)

Important Note: People with back problems should consult their doctor before doing this exercise.

Instructions:

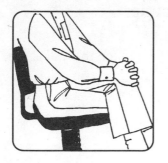

1. Sitting comfortably in a chair (with thighs higher than knees) and with both feet on the floor, cross your left leg over your right, clasp your hands together on your left knee and interlock your fingers.

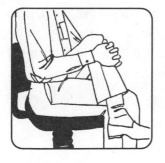

2. Using your arms pull your left leg up and to the right (diagonally across your body). Keep your body straight. Hold for 30 seconds. Feel the stretch in your lower back and alongside the outer part of your left thigh.

REPEAT once with the right leg.

Notes:
- Go slowly and lift your leg up with only your arms and only as far as comfortable.
- Relax your legs and hips.
- Breathe regularly and easily.

NEAR TO FAR SHIFTING: 1 EYE

Purpose: To regain flexibility in the extraocular muscles (that control eye movements) and increase the ease with which your eyes change focus.

POSITION	REPETITIONS	TIME
Seated	5 times (each eye)	1 1/2 minutes

Materials: Pen or pencil
Optional materials: Eye patch

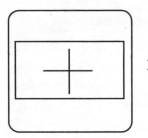

Set up:

1. Place the + Chart (P. 143) on the wall at eye level when seated.

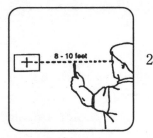

2. Sit 8 to 10 feet away. Hold a pen (or pencil) in your left hand at arm's length. Focus on the pen point or on a letter or mark printed on the pen. Be sure you have a clear, sharp focus.

Instructions:

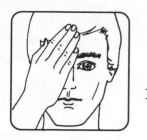

1. Cover your right eye with the palm of your right hand, being careful not to touch your eye/eyelid. (Or, if you have an eye patch, use it.) Keep the covered eye open, too.

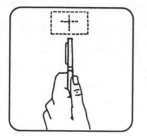

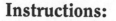

2. With your left eye, look at the pen point (or the letter or mark) and bring it into focus. Hold your focus for 3 to 5 seconds. Blink and breathe.

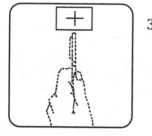

3. Now, shift your focus from the pen point/letter/mark to the far target and bring it into focus. Again, hold for 3 to 5 seconds. Blink and breathe. Shift back and forth four more times, focusing on each target for 3 to 5 seconds.

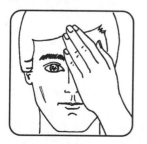

REPEAT steps 2 and 3
with your left eye covered, but open.

Notes:

- Do not continue to shift when the image you are focusing on is blurred. Make sure that you bring it into focus and see it clearly before you shift your vision (again). Blinking will help you maintain focus and clarity.
- Blink lightly and often, breathe regularly and easily, make sure your posture is correct and relaxed, and be aware of objects in your peripheral vision. This cannot be emphasized enough.
- Avoid any temptation to go faster. Rushing is a sign of poor eye control and symptomatic of an attitude that "wants to get it over with." Actually, the real need is to relax and be patient. Stay in the moment.
- Initially, you may notice that it's easier, more natural and more spontaneous shifting in one of the directions. As you continue to practice you will develop equal ease, speed and comfort shifting in both directions.
- Also, as your skill improves move the pen progressively closer to your eyes. Do this gradually (over a period of weeks) until you can hold the pen 10 inches from your eyes and still shift comfortably..i).Exercises:Near to Far Shifting:1 eye;

NEAR TO FAR SHIFTING: 2 EYES

Purpose: To improve eye coordination and help develop the balanced use of both eyes.

POSITION	REPETITIONS	TIME
Seated	5 times	30 seconds

Materials: Pen or pencil

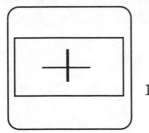

Set up:

1. Place the + Chart (P. 143) on the wall at eye level when seated.

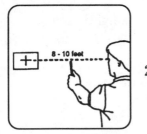

2. Sit 8 to 10 feet away. Hold a pen (or pencil) in your left hand at arms length. Focus on the pen point (or on a letter or mark on the pen). Be sure you have a clear, sharp focus.

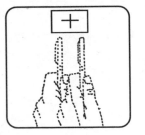

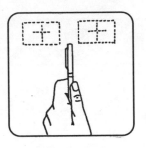

Instructions:

1. As you focus on the letter, mark or pen point with both eyes, in the background see the illusion of two images of the far chart. Hold for 2 breaths. Blink.

2. Now shift your focus to the far chart. In the foreground, see the illusion of two pens. Hold for 2 breaths. Blink lightly and often.

REPEAT 4 times.

Notes:

- Make sure that you shift your focus in a relaxed and easy manner. Do not rush.

- Make sure that your focus goes **all the way** to each target and rests on it for 2 breaths before shifting back to the other target.

- If you see only one pen or one target (instead of two), make sure both eyes are open, that you're seated *directly* in front of the target, and that the pen is in front of you between you and the target.

- If you don't see two images or begin to lose the illusion of the two, either near or far, close your eyes and take a deep breath. Then reopen your eyes, blink lightly and often, breathe regularly and deeply, and open up your peripheral awareness.

- If you still see only one target (or one pen) it means that your mind is blocking out or suppressing the image from one eye. To help activate the mind's use of both your eyes try issuing a verbal command such as, "Mind, use both eyes equally," or "See two pens," etc. Or make up your own command.

- Initially, you may notice that it's easier, more natural and more spontaneous shifting in one direction. As you continue to practice you will develop equal ease, speed and comfort shifting in both directions.

- As your ease, speed and comfort shifting in both directions increases, gradually hold the pen closer to your nose until you can hold the pen 3 to 5 inches from your nose and still have the ability to easily shift and see two images.

OCCIPITAL POINT MASSAGE

Purpose: To stimulate acupressure points in the occipital region and reduce neck tension.

POSITION	REPETITIONS	TIME
Seated or standing	2 times (each side)	40 seconds

Instructions:

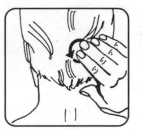

1. Find the occipital acupressure points by following the muscles on either sides of your spine up the back of your neck to where they meet the base of the skull. The points that are most tender or sensitive are the ones you want to massage.

2. As you inhale, apply deep (but not painful) pressure with both fingertips. Rotate your fingertips in small circles as you apply this pressure for 10 seconds on both the left and the right sides. Exhale as you release the pressure.

REPEAT one time.

Notes:
- Keep your eyes open throughout this exercise.

PALMING

Purpose: To relax tired and strained eyes, restore peace and quiet to your mind and provide much-needed rejuvenation.

POSITION	REPETITIONS	TIME
Seated	for 3 deep breaths	20 - 30 seconds

Instructions:

1. Briskly rub your hands and palms together for 5 to 10 seconds until they are warm.

2. Cup your warmed palms over your *closed* eyes. Relax your brow. As you exhale, imagine letting go of the tension from your eyes. Breathe regularly and easily.

Notes:

- The fingers of each hand should overlap and rest gently on the center of your forehead. Do not touch your closed eyes/eyelids or put pressure on your nose.
- Sparks, dots of light or patterns of color are signs that you are releasing mental strain and nervous tension.
- Seeing blackness with your eyes closed indicates visual relaxation. As your eyes become more and more relaxed, the black will appear even more black.
- If your arms get tired, rest your elbows on a desktop or on your thighs.

SHOULDER SHRUGS/ROTATIONS

Purpose: To reduce shoulder tension, neck tension and relax the upper body.

POSITION	REPETITIONS	TIME
Standing	5 times (each exercise)	1 minute

SHOULDER SHRUGS

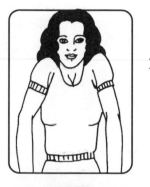

Instructions:

1. Inhale fully and deeply and lift both shoulders up as high as you can. Hold your shoulders up high and tight and hold your breath for a count of five.

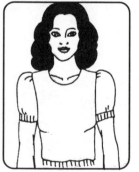

2. Now, exhale quickly and completely, letting your shoulders drop all at once, as if you were throwing them down.

REPEAT 4 times.

SHOULDER ROTATIONS

Instructions:

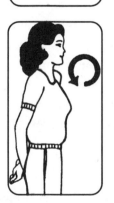

1. Grasp your left wrist with your right hand behind your back. Drop your shoulders and let them relax.

2. On the inhale, *very slowly* rotate both shoulders forward, then upward towards your ears (clockwise). As you exhale, continue rotating your shoulders back and around to the starting position.

REPEAT 4 times.

Notes:
- Go *very slowly* with this movement. Over time you will become more limber.

TEMPLE/EYE MASSAGE

Purpose: To stimulate the acupressure points associated with good vision and reduce eyestrain and facial tension.

POSITION	REPETITIONS	TIME
Seated or standing	8 times (each of the 6 parts)	60-75 seconds

Set up: Wash your hands before doing these exercises.

Instructions:

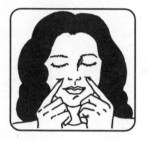

1. With your fingertips locate a point about two fingertips from the sides of your nostrils and in a vertical line from your pupils. Stimulate this point by pressing deeply for 1 second and releasing the pressure for 1 second. (Deep pressure means feeling aching pain on the pressured point, which disappears when you release the pressure.) Inhale as you apply pressure and exhale on the release. **REPEAT 7 times.**

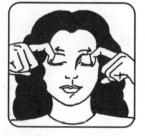

2. Place the sides of both (bent) index fingers against the top of your nose feeling for the inside of your eye sockets. (IMPORTANT: Do not press on or against your eyeball!) Now, applying deep pressure, draw your fingers along the inner edges of the top of your eye sockets. Draw your fingers outward, from your nose toward your temples, inhaling on the pressured movement, exhaling on the release. **REPEAT 7 times.**

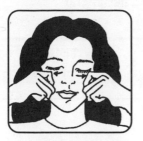

3. Now, draw your bent fingers along the inner edges of the bottom of your eye sockets. Inhale as you apply pressure and exhale on the release. **REPEAT 7 times.**

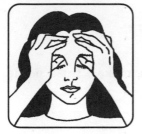

4. Place the tips of your fingers along your forehead and the tips of your thumbs under the inside corner of each eye socket. Locate the tender spot and apply deep upward pressure. Inhale on the pressure and exhale on the release. **REPEAT 7 times.**

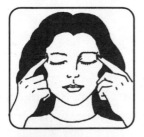

5. With the tips of your index fingers find the soft spots at the outer edges of your eyebrows. Feel for the most tender spot. Press for 1 second, then relax. Inhale on the pressure, exhale on the release. **REPEAT 7 times.**

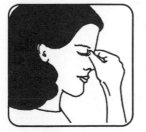

6. Using your thumb and index finger apply deep pressure to the inner corners of each eye. Press for 1 second, then relax. Inhale on the pressure, exhale on the release. **REPEAT 7 times.**

Notes:
- Keep your eyes closed during all of these exercises.

THUMB ROTATIONS

Purpose: To develop smooth and fluid eye movements, gain greater control of eye movements and expand peripheral awareness.

POSITION	REPETITIONS	TIME
Standing	5 rotations (each eye, in each direction)	2 minutes

Optional Material: Eye patch

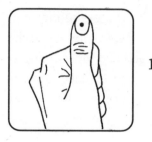

Set up:

1. With an erasable pen, make a small dot in the center of both thumbnails.

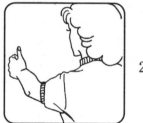

2. Extend your left hand arm's length, fingers gently curled into a relaxed fist, with your thumb pointing up.

Instructions:

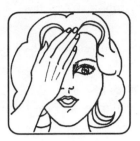

1. Cover your right eye with the palm of your right hand. Keep the palmed eye open.

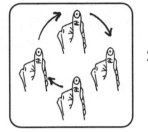

2. Keeping your left arm fully extended, thumb at eye level, move your thumb in a clockwise rotating circle, following the dot on your thumb with your eye. Blink and breathe. Follow the dot for 5 rotations.

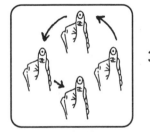

3. Repeat in a counterclockwise direction, following the dot for 5 rotations. Remember, blink and breathe.

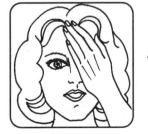

4. Cover the left eye with your left hand and repeat steps 2 and 3.

Notes:

- While the size of the circle is not important, it's better to start out small. Adjust your arm's movement to the ease of your eye's ability to follow comfortably and keep focus. It's important to do this exercise *slowly*.
- Be sure to make smooth eye movements in *all* directions, free of jumps.
- Make sure that your thumb always stays in focus, too.
- Peripheral awareness and background awareness are also important. Keep your eye on the dot and increase your awareness of the periphery, thereby opening up your visual awareness.
- As you practice this technique you may notice that your ability to maintain focus on the dot will increase, as will your awareness and clarity of the objects in your peripheral vision.

Part Two

ENHANCING YOUR VISION

HOW YOUR EYES WORK AT THE COMPUTER: CRITICAL VISUAL SKILLS

It is a commonly held belief that clear distance sight without glasses constitutes "perfect vision." While this certainly is desirable, there are many other components to vision, among them the abilities to maintain efficient visual performance and clear comfortable vision at the computer for an extended period of time.

To maintain clear and relaxed focus at the computer for an extended period of time your eyes have to make a sustained adjustment of focus and perform a precise set of repetitive, coordinated movements.

There are six distinct abilities that your visual system must possess to perform effectively and efficiently at the computer. We call them the Critical Visual Skills. They are accommodation, convergence, saccadic movement, pursuit movement, peripheral awareness and cognitive awareness.

Efficient visual performance at the computer is much more complex than simply sharpness of vision. In fact, efficient close-up visual performance requires *all* six of the Critical Visual Skills.

Let's look at them.

Accommodation is the ability of your eyes to change focus. A group of muscles inside each eye — the ciliary body — controls this ability *(Fig. 5)*. As long as you look at the screen, the ciliary body must hold your focus at a fixed and unchanging distance. If it "lets go," your focus changes and the screen becomes blurred. If it "cramps," your vision becomes blurred when you look into the distance, or you experience sluggishness in shifting your focus from near to far.

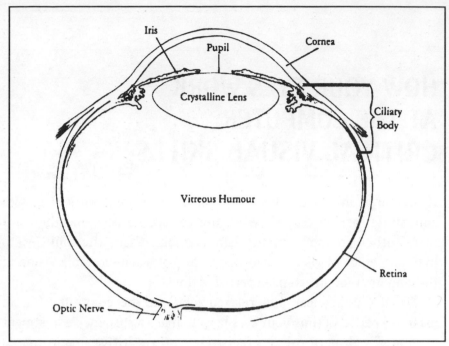

Fig. 5   The ciliary body is a group of muscles that controls the ability of your eyes to change focus.

Convergence is the ability to use both eyes together. Convergence requires a series of coordinated movements of the muscles of both eyes. Six muscles around each eye — the extraocular muscles — control pointing and movements of the eyes *(Fig. 6)*. One task of these muscles is to point both eyes at the same spot on the screen at the same time.

The extraocular muscles also perform a series of precise, repetitive movements as you read from the screen or input into the computer. These are called **saccadic movements**. A related skill of the extraocular muscles is **pursuit movement**, which is the ability of the eyes to follow a moving object smoothly.

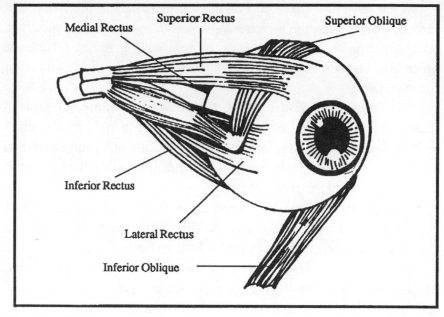

Fig. 6   Six extraocular muscles control pointing and movements of the eyes.

The eyes are not actually supported by the extraocular muscles, only directed by them, so there is no need for great strength. Nevertheless, the muscles are several hundred times stronger than they need to be. Eye turns and associated vision problems are not caused by muscle weakness, but by a lack of learned control.

Since the eyes are in constant movement, it is not likely that these muscles will cramp the way the ciliary muscles can. However, tension in the extraocular muscles can cause rigidity and inflexibility in eye movements as well as a feeling of fatigue. Fatigue and tension in the extraocular muscles may take several forms: eyestrain, headache, loss of attention or concentration, blurred or double vision, or a general feeling of irritability.

The ultimate purpose of vision is to provide information to the brain. This requires a high degree of coordination between your eyes and your brain. Thus, the active involvement of the brain in seeing at the computer is just as important as the active involvement of the muscles that control the focusing of the eyes and eye movements.

At the same time that your eyes are focused on a specific area of the screen, images from the periphery enter your eyes — also registering on the retina. The brain needs to maintain a balance between processing visual information from the center of your vision and from the periphery.

The fifth Critical Visual Skill is the ability to use, in an organized manner, your **peripheral awareness**. Concentrating intently on a small area of the screen (and thereby mentally blocking out your peripheral awareness) can result in mental fatigue and a decline in both concentration and performance.

In addition, the brain has to process, integrate and understand all the visual information it receives. The sixth Critical Visual Skill, **cognitive awareness**, is so basic that it is often overlooked.

Your eyes "see" only the letters C - A - T. It is the total visual process that produces the image of a cat in your mind. The more abstract the information, the greater the demands on the resources of the brain.

Extended periods of concentration and mental effort — e.g., computer work — can surface deficiencies in your visual processing system with the resulting symptoms of double or blurred vision, reduced performance, or mental fatigue and strain.

Shortcomings in Critical Visual Skill fitness are usually not evident until you experience the kinds of discomforts and stresses that have led you to this book.

The Vision Enhancement Training in this section will sharpen your Critical Visual Skills and get your entire visual system into the shape it needs to be in to meet the rigorous visual demands of computer work.

GETTING YOUR VISION IN SHAPE: VISION ENHANCEMENT TRAINING

The greater the overall fitness of your visual system, the longer you will be able to work at a computer *without* experiencing any of the visual symptoms of Computer Stress Syndrome.

Conversely, if your visual system is not in the best shape, you will be more prone to fatigue, discomfort, eyestrain and focusing problems.

This Vision Enhancement Training will get the critical parts of your vision into the condition necessary for sustained computer work.

How it works

The Vision Enhancement Training takes about 15-20 minutes.

Practice the entire routine daily or practice 2 or 3 exercises a day, cycling through the entire routine every 3 or 4 days.

Either way, continue using the routine until all the exercises can be performed easily and effortlessly.

After that, use the routine 2 or 3 times a week to maintain your vision at its maximum level.

General guidelines for all exercises

When practicing any of the Vision Enhancement Training exercises always remember the basic guidelines:

- Maintain good posture
- Breathe regularly and easily
- Blink lightly and often
- Keep your body as relaxed as possible
- Make all movements slow and smooth
- Keep a relaxed mental attitude

(See Pp. 49-50 for more information about these guidelines.)

Vision Enhancement Training Summary		
EXERCISE	**REPETITIONS**	*CRITICAL VISUAL SKILL*
PENCIL AWARENESS	1 minute	*Peripheral Awareness*
PENCIL TRACKING	5 rotations (each eye, in each direction)	*Pursuit Movement*
WALL FIXATIONS	6 times (each way)	*Saccadic Movement*
CHART TO CHART	5 times (each eye)	*Accommodation*
FUSION STRING	3 times (up and down the string)	*Convergence*
CHART TO CHART: READING ALOUD:	5 times (each eye)	*Cognitive Awareness*
PERIPHERAL CHART	2 times	*Peripheral Awareness*

CRITICAL VISUAL SKILL: PERIPHERAL AWARENESS

PENCIL AWARENESS

Purpose: To expand the range of your peripheral awareness and develop greater relaxation while concentrating.

POSITION	REPETITIONS	TIME
Standing	- -	1 minute

Materials: Two pencils

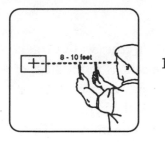

Set up:

1. Stand directly in front of a visual target (a clock, a calendar, etc.) that is eye height on a wall 8 to 10 feet away. Hold a pencil in each hand in front of each eye.

Instructions:

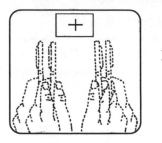

1. Focus on the wall target. In the foreground, see two images of each pencil. Blink and breathe.

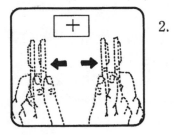

2. Keeping focused on the wall target, gradually move the pencils to the sides of your vision. Maintain your awareness of the four images until the pencils are too far apart to see the four images. Then, move the pencils in random directions — in and out, back and forth — the whole time keeping your focus on the wall target and maintaining your awareness of the four images of the pencils. Do this for 1 minute.

Notes:
- If you lose awareness of the double images, close your eyes, take a deep breath, then reopen your eyes and continue.
- Remember to blink lightly and often, to keep your body relaxed, and to breathe regularly and easily.
- It is helpful to have color contrast between the pencils and the wall target (i.e., dark pencils and light background) and the target should have good contrast against the wall as well.

CRITICAL VISUAL SKILL: PURSUIT MOVEMENT

PENCIL TRACKING

Purpose: To develop smooth and fluid eye movements and enhance control of eye movements.

POSITION	REPETITIONS	TIME
Standing	5 rotations (each eye, in each direction)	2 minutes

Materials: Pencil (or pen) with a small dot marked on it
Optional Materials: Eye patch

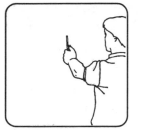

Set up:

1 . Hold the pencil at arm's length in your left hand.

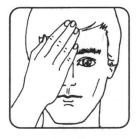

Instructions (Level One):

1. Cover your right eye with the palm of your right hand or an eye patch. Keep the covered eye open.

2. Keeping your left arm fully extended, slowly move the pencil in a clockwise circle, centered at eye level. Look at the mark on the pencil, following the rotation with your eye. Blink and breathe. Follow the mark for a total of 5 rotations.

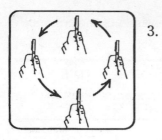

3. Repeat slowly, in a counter-clockwise direction for 5 rotations, too. Remember to blink and breathe.

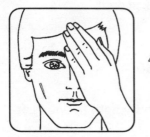

4. Repeat with your left eye covered with your left hand (or eye patch).

Notes:
- While the size of the circle is not important, it's better to start out small. Adjust your arm's movement to the ease of your eye's ability to follow comfortably and keep focus. Again, it is important to do this exercise *slowly*.
- Be sure to make smooth eye movements in *all* directions, free of jumps.
- Make sure that your thumb always stays in focus, too.
- Peripheral awareness and background awareness are important. Keep your eye on the mark and maintain awareness of the periphery.
- As you practice this technique you will notice that your ability to maintain focus on the mark will increase as will your awareness and clarity of the objects in your peripheral vision.

Once you are comfortable with Level One, move on to the next three levels:

Instructions (Level Two):

Follow the mark on the pencil as you move it randomly — in and out, up and down, and diagonally.

Instructions (Level Three):

Repeat Level Two except follow the mark on the pencil with your eyes *closed*. Occasionally, open your eyes to be sure that you are, indeed, following the pencil.

Instructions (Level Four):

Instead of completely blocking out the covered eye, use just two fingers to obstruct the view of the pencil. This will permit you to maintain peripheral awareness with that eye. Notice what you observe and what you can see as you move the pencil.

CRITICAL VISUAL SKILL: SACCADIC MOVEMENT

WALL FIXATIONS

Purpose: To develop smooth eye movements and greater muscular coordination between the movements of both eyes.

POSITION	REPETITIONS	TIME
Standing	6 times	1 minute

Materials: Ten 3x5 index cards and a felt-tipped pen
Optional Materials: Eye patch

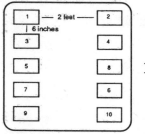

Set up:

1. Write the numbers from 1 to 10 on ten index cards and then mount the cards on the wall in two columns 2 feet apart with the cards in each column 6-8 inches apart. Make sure the room is well lit and that there is no glare on the cards.

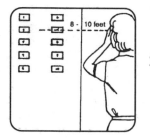

2. Stand 8 to 10 feet from the wall.

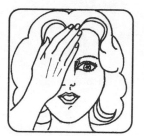

Instructions (Level One):

1. Cover your left eye with your left hand (or an eye patch), but keep it open.

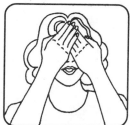

2. Starting at number 1, shift your focus rhythmically and consecutively from number to number at about one shift per second all the way to number 10. Blink and breathe and be aware of your peripheral vision.

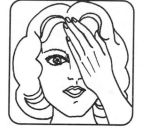

3. When you finish the first 10, close both eyes and palm as you breathe deeply 4 times. Relax your brow.

4. Now, repeat this with your right eye covered but open.

REPEAT 5 times.

Notes:
- Remember to stand correctly and comfortably and to keep your head straight and not tilted or turned.
- As always, blink, breathe and be aware of your peripheral vision.

Once you are comfortable going from 1 to 10 in a rhythmic way, move on to the next two levels:

Instructions (Level Two):

Practice the exercise starting at number 10 and moving backwards — rhythmically — to number 1.

Instructions (Level Three):

Once you are comfortable going from 1 to 10 forwards and backwards, rearrange the numbers on the wall in a random pattern, and continue to shift rhythmically in numerical order.

CRITICAL VISUAL SKILL: ACCOMMODATION

CHART TO CHART SHIFTING

Purpose: To exercise, tone and increase the flexibility of the extraocular muscles and to make changing focus smoother and easier.

POSITION	REPETITIONS	TIME
Seated	5 times (each eye)	60 - 75 seconds

Materials: Small and Large Letter Charts
Optional Materials: Eye patch

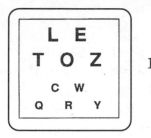

Set up:

1. Mount the Large Letter Chart (P. 147) on the wall so that it's at eye level when seated.

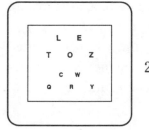

2. You'll also use the Small Letter Chart (P. 149), but bring it to your seat.

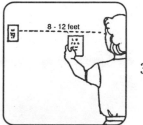

3. Sit 8-12 feet from the Large Letter Chart and hold the Small Letter Chart in your left hand at arm's length.

Instructions:

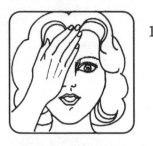

1. Cover your right eye with the palm of your right hand or an eye patch. Again, keep the covered eye open.

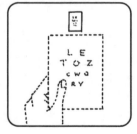

2. Pick a letter on the Small Letter Chart in your hand, focus on it, see it clearly, then shift your vision to the same letter on the Large Letter Chart, focus on it and see it clearly. Continue shifting, back and forth, from near to far at a rate of approximately one letter per second. Count "*1 Mississippi, 2 Mississippi,*" etc., until you have shifted through all 10 letters. Remember to blink lightly and often, breathe, and be aware of the periphery.

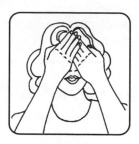

3. When you are finished with the left eye, palm over both closed eyes for 10-15 seconds. *(See Palming exercise on P. 85.)*

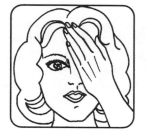

4. Then, repeat with your left eye covered and open.

REPEAT 4 times.

Notes:

- Make sure that both charts are well lit and without glare.
- Try to achieve a quick clearing of the chart at the moment of shifting.
- Blink lightly and often, breathe regularly and easily, make sure your posture is correct and relaxed, and maintain an awareness of your peripheral vision.
- As you progress, bring the Small Letter Chart closer to your eyes until it is 3 to 5 inches away.

CRITICAL VISUAL SKILL: CONVERGENCE

FUSION STRING TECHNIQUE

Purpose: To develop convergence — the ability of both eyes to look at the same point at the same time.

POSITION	REPETITIONS	TIME
Standing	3 times (up and down the string)	1 1/2 to 2 minutes

Materials: Fusion String

(You can make your own Fusion String by stringing 10 beads on a six-foot-long string with the beads about six inches apart. Or you can get a Fusion String from the Cambridge Institute for Better Vision, 65 Wenham Road, Topsfield, MA 01983. Please include $3.00 for postage and handling.)

Set up:

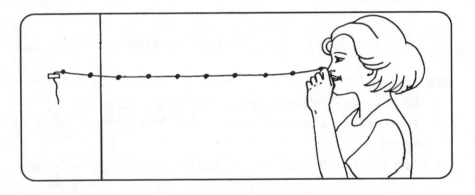

1. Attach one end of the Fusion String to the wall with a piece of tape or a push pin at a height slightly lower than eye level when standing. Good illumination is critical. Wrap the free end of the Fusion String around your index finger and hold the string up to the tip of your nose. The string should make a straight but slightly downward line from your nose to the wall. ***Do not lean forward or tilt backwards to make the string straight***. Instead, step a little closer to, or farther away from, the wall.

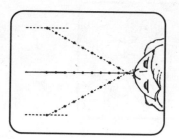

Instructions:

1. First, look at your nose and see the illusion of two strings meeting in a "V" at your nose. Blink, breathe and use your peripheral vision.

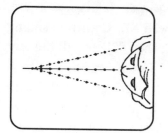

2. Now, shift your gaze to the wall at where the string attaches. Again, see the illusion of two strings meeting in a "V" at the wall.

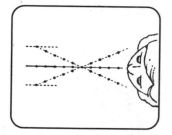

3. Next, shift your vision to bead #5 and see the illusion of two strings crossing in an "X" over bead #5, with the center of the "X" directly on bead #5.

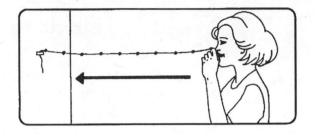

4 . Now slide your gaze to bead #1 (closest to nose) and focus on it. The illusion of the two strings meeting in an "X" is now there, with the center of the "X" directly on bead #1. Continue sliding your gaze down the string — to bead #2, then #3, etc., all the way to bead #10 (closest to wall), focusing on each bead and at each bead seeing the illusion of the two strings meeting in an "X," with the center of the "X" directly on the bead at which you are looking. After you finish bead #10, look at the wall and see the illusion of two strings meeting in a "V" at the wall.

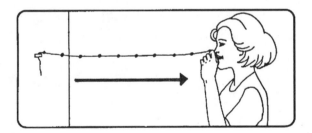

5. Now, reverse direction, starting at bead #10, to bead #9, then #8, etc., all the way to bead #1 (closest to nose). After you finish bead #1, look at your nose and again see the illusion of two strings meeting there.

REPEAT 2 times.

Notes:

- Sometimes, instead of seeing the "X" directly on the bead people see:
  - * two strings crossing in an "X," but the strings are either crossing beyond or in front of the bead;
  - * two strings crossing at some point and continuing in one string, so a "Y" is seen rather than an "X;"
  - * two strings that do not cross at all;
  - * only one string instead of two;
  - * one string more solidly than the other. (To learn which eye is seeing, alternately close each eye and notice which string disappears.)

- If you notice any of the above: blink lightly and often, breathe regularly and easily, make sure your posture is relaxed, and open up your peripheral vision.

- As you move your eyes up and down the string, *slide* your gaze along the string from bead to bead instead of jumping. Also, pay most attention to the crossover areas — the places where the "X" stops following the commands of your mind.

- For example, say you are able to make the "X" cross at beads #1, #2, #3 and #4, but when you look at bead #5 the "X" seems to stay stuck at bead #4. If this happens, then slide your gaze back and forth over the "crossover point" between beads #4 and #5. (You might also go up to bead #6 and work your way back to #5.) Eventually, sliding your gaze back and forth will help relieve the stuckness. Always work toward sliding the "X" further away from you *or* closer to you, whichever the direction of improvement.

- At first, you might find it easier to start at the further beads and slide your gaze in towards your nose. With practice, it will become easier to move in either direction with equal ease and comfort.
- Issuing spoken or silent verbal commands from your mind to your eyes when your eyes do not place the "X" where you want it will help to accelerate your progress. Simple commands such as "Eyes, focus where I tell you," "Eyes, look at where my mind wants you to," and "See the 'X'," are effective. Experiment. Make up your own commands.
- At first improvement may not come in the form of clarity but in your being able to see the "X" and move the "X" *under your control* within larger and larger areas.

CRITICAL VISUAL SKILL: COGNITIVE AWARENESS

CHART TO CHART SHIFTING: READING ALOUD

Purpose: To integrate visual and cognitive skills and to develop more efficient mental processing of visual information.

POSITION	REPETITIONS	TIME
Standing	5 times (each eye)	60 - 75 seconds

Materials: Small and Large Letter Chart.
Optional Materials: Eye patch

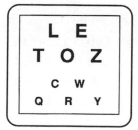

Set up:

1. Mount the Large Letter Chart (P. 147) on the wall so that it is at eye level when seated.

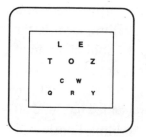

2. Bring the Small Letter Chart (P. 149) to your seat.

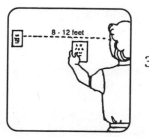

3. Sit 8-12 feet from the Large Letter Chart and hold the Small Letter Chart in your left hand at arm's length.

Instructions:

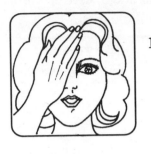

1. Cover your right eye with the palm of your right hand (or an eye patch). Keep the covered eye open.

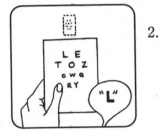

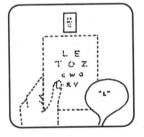

2. Pick a letter on the Small Letter Chart in your hand, focus on it, and call it out loud as you see it clearly, then shift your vision to the same letter on the Large Letter Chart, focus on it and call it out loud as you see it clearly. Continue shifting, back and forth, from near to far, calling each letter out loud as you shift to it. Shift at a rate of approximately one letter per second (count "*1 Mississippi, 2 Mississippi,*" etc.) until you have shifted through and called out loud all 10 letters. Remember to blink lightly and often, breathe regularly and easily, and be aware of the periphery.

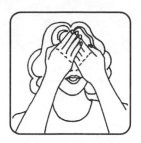

3. When you are finished with the left eye, palm over both *closed* eyes for 10-15 seconds. (See Palming exercise on P. 85.)

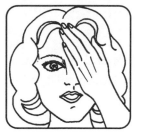

4. Then, repeat with your left eye covered and open.

REPEAT 4 times.

Notes:
- Make sure that both charts are well lit and without glare.
- Call out the letter *at the same time* that you shift to it, rather than slightly before or after.
- Try to achieve a quick clearing of the chart at the moment of shifting.
- Blink lightly and often, breathe regularly and easily, make sure your posture is correct and relaxed, and maintain an awareness of your peripheral vision.
- As you progress, bring the Small Letter Chart closer to your eyes until it is 3 to 5 inches away.

CRITICAL VISUAL SKILL: PERIPHERAL AWARENESS

PERIPHERAL AWARENESS CHART

Purpose: To expand the range of your peripheral awareness and develop greater relaxation while concentrating intently on a visual task.

POSITION	REPETITIONS	TIME
Standing	2 times	30 - 45 seconds

Set up:

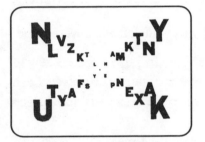

1. Attach the Peripheral Awareness Chart (P. 134) to the wall at eye level when standing. (Or, you can hold the chart in your hand at eye level.)

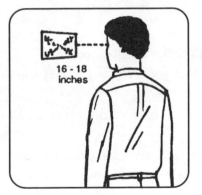

16 - 18 inches

2. Stand 16-18 inches from the chart.

Instructions:

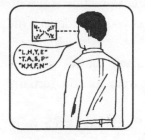

1. Focus on the letter in the center of the chart. Without moving your eyes, call out the letters on the first ring. Continue looking at the center letter as you call out the letters in each successive ring. Blink and breathe and be aware of your periphery.

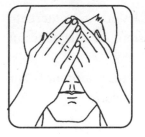

2. When you have read as many letters as you can, close your eyes and palm over both eyes. Relax your brow as you take 3 deep breaths.

REPEAT one more time.

Notes:

- Through the repetition of regular and consistent practice you will be able to call out *all* the letters on the chart as you stay focused on the letter in the center.
- As your peripheral awareness expands, you will notice certain letters on the chart become clearer and sharper as you remain focused on the letter in the center.
- Make sure that you are standing correctly (P. 51) and keep your head straight and not tilted or turned.
- You may find it helpful — before calling out letters — to increase your mental awareness of your peripheral vision, i.e., the edges of the card.
- If you use glasses or contacts, try doing this exercise *without* them — it will be better training for your peripheral vision.

Part Three

ELECTROMAGNETIC FIELDS (EMFs) AND THE COMPUTER

ELECTROMAGNETIC FIELDS (EMFs): HARMLESS OR HAZARDOUS?

Ever since computers made their large-scale appearance in the workplace in the mid-70s the most-often asked question has been: "Are emissions from electromagnetic fields from video display terminals a health hazard?"

The answer depends on whom you ask:

Yale physicist: "There are very good reasons to believe that weak ELF (extremely low frequency) fields can have no significant biological effects — and no strong reason to believe otherwise."[1]

Computer industry lobbyist: "For pregnant operators to ask to be transferred away from video display terminals (VDTs) 'is like asking to be transferred away from a light bulb.'"[2]

MacWorld editor: "Extremely-low-frequency (ELF) magnetic emissions may prove to be one of the most troublesome issues we face with information technology over the next decade..."[3]

Boston Globe internal memo to employees: "The medical department feels that there is sufficient reason to take steps to reduce exposure..."[4]

After more than 50 investigations in the United States, Canada and Europe over the last 16 years there is still no consensus of opinion — either in the scientific community or in the computer industry — that there is or isn't a health hazard from video display terminals.

Basis of the debate

Video display terminals produce images on the screen through an internal "picture tube" called a cathode ray tube (CRT). These tubes emit electromagnetic fields at two frequencies: very low frequencies (VLF) and extremely low frequencies (ELF). Both VLF and ELF fields are each made up of electric and magnetic components. These electromagnetic emissions occur whenever the VDT is turned on (even if the screen's brightness control is turned down).

VLF and ELF are only two forms of electromagnetic emissions. Others include radio and TV waves, microwaves, X-rays and nuclear radiation.

Scientists do agree that some electromagnetic emissions have been proven to be highly dangerous (nuclear radiation); other emissions pose no known health hazard (TV and radio waves); and still others, we are told to restrict our exposure to (microwave, X-rays).

The ELFs coming from VDTs are similar in nature to the type that emanate from electric blankets, toaster ovens, hair dryers and other common household electrical devices. The difference, contend those who believe EMFs may be dangerous, is that people spend 8-12 hours a day in front of computer screens — within distances where emissions measure highest.

The heart of the controversy depends on whether you consider these emissions to be safe until proven hazardous or hazardous until proven safe. Therein lies the debate.

Cause for concern?

It started in 1977 when two copy editors at *The New York Times* — working on VDTs for a year or less — developed cataracts. They claimed that the cataracts were "radiation induced." Five years later, the Panel on Impact of Video Viewing on Vision of Workers found "no scientifically valid evidence that occupational use of VDTs is associated with increased risk of ocular diseases or abnormalities, including cataracts."[5]

Between 1979 and 1984, the controversy escalated when eleven different clusters of birth defects and miscarriages involving women who worked at VDTs were reported in the U.S. and Canada. (A "cluster" is an occurrence of two or more similar phenomena [i.e., miscarriages and birth defects] in a particular situation [i.e., computers in a single location].) Further studies, however, seemed to indicate that these clusters could not be definitively linked to VDTs.[6] The debate continues.

Similar reports of clusters of birth defects and/or miscarriages have since been reported in Great Britain, Sweden, Australia and Denmark.

Research and epidemiological studies

During 1980 and 1981, Dr. José M.R. Delgado, a neurophysicist and director of research at Centro Ramón y Cajal Hospital in Madrid, Spain, and Jocelyne Leal, a cell biologist, investigated the biological effects of weak pulsed ELF magnetic fields — similar to the kind emanating from VDTs — on chick embryos. They discovered that nearly 80 percent of the embryos had developed abnormally.[7]

In 1984, scientists at the Swedish National Board of Occupational Safety and Health confirmed these findings. But in 1985, Professor Arthur W. Guy, director of the Bioelectromagnetic Research Laboratory at the University of Washington in Seattle, dismissed the conclusions because the weak magnetic-field pulses used by Delgado and Leal, though similar, did not "match the pulses emitted by computer display monitors."[8]

In 1987, Dr. Hakon Frölen, of the Swedish University of Agricultural Sciences, linked VDT-type fields with abnormal pregnancies in mice. Frölen's experiments "found a significant increase in fetal death and fetal losses by resorption (a phenomenon similar to miscarriage in humans) among pregnant mice exposed to weak pulsed magnetic fields."[9]

A word of caution: What is true for mice and chickens may not be true for human beings. Different studies which rely on animal models and which produce conflicting results are far from definitive proof of any hazard to humans.

Because direct experimentation on human subjects is — of course — not permitted, epidemiological studies are conducted for answers. But these studies have serious drawbacks.

An epidemiological study attempts to associate different risk factors with specific groups of people. But even if there is a positive outcome the association is statistical and not necessarily causal. For example, if a connection between VDTs and health were established, it might be a result of postural factors or electromagnetic fields arising from building wiring rather than the computer, or any of a number of other factors. It is very difficult to isolate the exact nature of the cause.

One major reproductive epidemiological study in the U.S. was conducted by Kaiser Permanente Medical Care, the nation's largest health maintenance organization, in Oakland, California, in 1981-1982. The finding was that women who used VDTs more than 20 hours a week during the first trimester had an 80 percent higher risk of early and late miscarriages than women who did similar work without VDTs.

In their report, released in 1988, Kaiser researchers concluded: "Our case-control study provides the first epidemiological evidence based on substantial numbers of pregnant VDT operators to suggest that high usage of VDTs may increase the risk of miscarriage."[10]

But other researchers had different interpretations of the data, suspecting stress or other factors.

Another epidemiological study, by NIOSH between 1983-86, of spontaneous abortions among 2,430 telephone operators who used cathode ray tube VDTs compared with those who used other display devices, found no increased risk of miscarriage in the cathode ray tube VDT user group. Here researchers concluded that VLF fields were not a risk factor. But no conclusion was reached regarding ELF fields.[11]

A new Finnish epidemiological study completed in 1992 — "the first to look at measured magnetic field exposure for VDT operators" — reported a "significant increase in the number of miscarriages."

VDT NEWS, the bimonthly "VDT Health and Safety Report," said this study, by Dr. Maila Hietanen, of the Institute of Occupational Health in Helsinki, Finland, in collaboration with Dr. Marja-Liisa Lindbohm, an epidemiologist at the Helsinki Institute, "did not reveal miscarriage risk when women were classified according to the number of hours they worked at a VDT — the method used in most past pregnancy studies."

"It's only when exposures are classified according to actual magnetic field exposures that you see an effect," Hietanen said. "VDT workers should not be worried, because newer models do not have high magnetic fields — only the older models have high fields," she said. "If your VDT meets MPR II guidelines, you need not be worried."[12]

The Swedish standards

Sweden was the first country to establish guidelines for electromagnetic emissions for video display terminals.

In 1986 Sweden's National Board of Measurement and Testing established the guidelines that have become the *de facto* standard for U.S. manufacturers of CRT monitors. These guidelines (called MPR I) covered VLF magnetic emissions, electrostatic emissions and x-radiation. Even more stringent guidelines (MPR II) followed in 1991, also covering alternating electric fields and ELF magnetic fields.[13]

Perhaps nothing demonstrates the profound complexity of the VDT emissions issue more than this: It is not even known whether Sweden's emissions standards are safe or not. Why? Because these standards, though widely recognized and voluntarily adhered to by some manufacturers, are based on current measuring technologies and *not on medical evidence*. "No scientific studies have proven which levels should be permitted. These standards may be unnecessarily restrictive or possibly not restrictive enough."[14] Until scientists can determine if exposure to radiation is unsafe, or if exposure at certain levels is safe, we won't know.

Taking action

Not everyone is standing still waiting for the scientific jury to reach it's verdict.

The New York City Public Schools, which purchases 6,000 to 7,000 monitors every year, has decided, as of 1992, to buy only monitors that meet a far stricter standard for ELF magnetic fields than the Swedish MPR II guidelines.[15]

In 1990, the New York Occupational Safety and Health Committee urged women who are pregnant — or trying to get pregnant — to transfer away from VDT work.[16] The last contract signed by the American Federation of State, County and Municipal Employees, which covers 140,000 New York City employees, allows pregnant VDT operators to transfer to non-computer jobs.[17]

CBS also has redesigned workplaces in New York and Chicago so that employees working at VDTs are three feet from the sides or backs of the nearest computer monitors.[18]

The Boston Globe, New England's largest daily newspaper, on the advice of its medical department, also instituted a three-foot minimum distance.

An April 2, 1991, letter to *Globe* employees from medical director Dr. Terrence O'Malley summarizes this confusing dilemma perfectly:

"There is little cause for concern. If there are adverse health effects from VDT fields (and this has not been shown) these are very small compared to the known health risks from smoking, driving without a seat belt, high blood pressure or elevated cholesterol."

Acknowledging research that has shown "magnetic fields can have effects on biological systems," he went on: "It is still not known" whether magnetic fields from VDTs are harmful because "there have been no conclusive studies showing such effects."

"The medical department feels, however, that there is sufficient reason to take steps to reduce exposure until such time that research establishes the absence of significant biological effects from VDT fields. It will be many years before this is clarified."[19]

Raising public awareness

In the summer of 1989, award-winning medical and science reporter Paul Brodeur — who first alerted Americans to the dangers of asbestos and microwave radiation — brought the EMF controversy into the open with his three-part series in *The New Yorker* magazine. The first piece was on power lines; the last on video display terminals.[20]

Another strong advocate for more concerted EMF research is Louis Slesin, Ph.D., founder and publisher of two watchdog publications based in New York City. Slesin's *Microwave News* was the first U.S. publication to report on José Delgado and Jocelyne Leal's research on weak pulsed magnetic fields.[21]

In 1991, Slesin called the lack of current research into EMFs "a national disgrace." He feels the same way in 1993. "What I find frustrating," Slesin said, "is that these terminals are everywhere; on everyone's desk, in every school, in every house...and we know very little about electromagnetic fields."[22]

Conclusion

To date, it certainly has not been proven that VDTs pose a health hazard. No definitive information exists that suggests that there are unsafe levels of exposure.

But perhaps it is time — after more than 16 years of inconclusive and conflicting studies — for the computer industry, the scientific community and the government to join together and make a serious attempt to determine the answer.

In the meantime, there are concrete steps that you can take to reduce your exposure to the ELF and VLF fields emanating from computer monitors (see next chapter).

As *MacWorld's* editor Jerry Borrell concludes in his bold commentary in *MacWorld*: "...In the end, if we prove to have jumped to a conclusion that's wrong — at least people won't have suffered. But if we're right, and if manufacturers take action, many of the millions of computer users may never have to fear the technology that they've come to rely upon."[23]

---

[1] Deborah Branscum, Column, Conspicuous Consumer, "Electromagnetic Update/The Controversy—and Research—Continues," *MacWorld*, October 1991, pp. 65-68.

[2] Paul Brodeur, "The Magnetic-Field Menace," *MacWorld*, July 1990, pp. 136-45.

[3] Jerry Borrell, Commentary, "Is Your Computer Killing You?/Industrial-Age Problems Give Way To Information-Age Problems," *MacWorld*, July 1990, pp. 23-26.

[4] *"The Boston Globe* Avoids EMFs," *VDT NEWS,* May/June 1991, p. 3.

[5] James LaRue, "Terminal Illnesses," *Wilson Library Bulletin*, September 1991, pp. 85-88.

[6] Louis Slesin, "VDT radiation: What's known, what isn't," *Columbia Journalism Review*, November/December 1984, pp. 40-41.

[7] Paul Brodeur, *"Currents of Death/Power Lines, Computer Terminals, and the Attempt to Cover Their Threat to Your Health,"* Simon & Schuster, 1989, pp. 266-68.

[8] Brodeur, "The Magnetic-Field Menace," p. 141.

[9] Ibid., p. 142.

[10] Ibid., p. 142.

[11] "NIOSH FInds No Increased Risk of Miscarriage," *VDT NEWS*, May/June 1991, p. 5.

[12] "Strong VDT Magnetic Fields May Cause Miscarriages," *VDT NEWS*, March/April 1992, pp. 1, 10 and "Finnish Pregnancy Study: EMF Risks at Lower Levels," *VDT NEWS*, May/June 1992, p. 3.

[13] To get a copy of the Swedish MPR I guidelines handbook, write to: SWEDAC (Swedish Board for Technical Accreditation), Box 878, S-501, 15 Boras, Sweden; FAX: (44-033) 10 13 92. Inquire about the cost.

[14] Alfred Poor, "CRT Radiation: A Glowing Concern?", *PC Magazine,* 30 June 1992, pp. 117-118.

[15] "NYC Public Schools Demand Low EMFs," *VDT NEWS*, January/February 1992, pp. 117-18.

[16] Diana Hembree, "Warning: Computing Can Be Hazardous To Your Health," *MacWorld*, January 1990, pp. 150-157.

[17] Ann Claire Greiner, "Terminal Hazards," *Technology Review*, February/March 1991, pp. 16-17.

[18] Ibid. p. 17.

[19] *VDT NEWS*, May/June 1991, p. 3.

[20] The series, "Annals of Radiation: The Hazards of Electromagnetic Fields," appeared in June and became the basis for the book, *"Currents of Death."*

[21] Brodeur, *"Currents of Death,"* pp. 301-305.

[22] Interview, May 3, 1993, with Louis Slesin; publishing *VDT NEWS* since 1984 and *Microwave News* since 1981 (P.O. Box 1799, Grand Central Station, New York NY 10163, 212-517-2802).

[23] Borrell, *MacWorld*, July 1990, p. 26.

HOW TO MINIMIZE YOUR EXPOSURE

Nobody knows for sure whether exposure to VDT electromagnetic emissions is harmless or hazardous.

Until there is a definitive answer, we recommend that you practice "prudent avoidance"[1] — wherever and whenever possible reducing your exposure.

Here are the five steps we suggest:

Sit up to 28 inches away from your computer screen.

Electromagnetic fields drop dramatically with distance. Sitting up to arm's length away from your screen reduces your EMF exposure from the front of the VDT. Fields are higher at 12 inches and increase as you get closer to the screen.[2]

Stay 4 to 5 feet away from the backs and sides of other monitors, laser printers and laser copiers.

Magnetic fields from the sides and backs of monitors are considerably stronger than those given off from the front.[3] Most likely, your greatest exposure is from other peoples' machines. If possible, rearrange how computers are set up in the office. Electromagnetic fields go through barriers, partitions and wall dividers, so only distance will reduce exposure.[4]

Turn off monitors when not in use.

Dimming the brightness control on the screen (or the use of a screen saver) **does not** reduce electromagnetic emissions.

Use a lower-emission monitor.

At least two dozen companies make monitors that meet Sweden's MPR II guidelines. But even if a monitor is called "low emission," it doesn't necessarily mean that it is in compliance with MPR II. You need to ask. (Safe Computing, Inc., 1-800-638-9121, can make your traditional monitor a low emission one.)

There are also many shielding devices — anti-radiation, anti-glare and anti-static screens — and while many profess to block all emissions, remember there is no external device for VDT monitors that blocks both electric and magnetic VLF and ELF fields.[5]

(Contact the Cambridge Institute, 1-800-372-3937, for a list of companies that offer low emission monitors.)

Use a Liquid Crystal Display (LCD) monitor.

LCD, gas plasma and electroluminescent screens (the type used for laptops) do not emit electromagnetic fields.[6] Perhaps a too-expensive alternative for some, this is the only sure way to avoid exposure.

Err on the side of caution

Sometime in the future it may turn out that these steps to reduce exposure will be shown to have been unnecessary. Or that "playing it safe" now on the side of caution was prudent on your part.

"The twenty-eight inches is a rule of thumb," says Slesin. "The idea is to put distance between you and your terminal." This, along with using a terminal that meets Sweden's MPR II guidelines, he says, "gives you more margins of safety."[7]

---

[1] Suzanne Stefanac, "At Arm's Length," MacWorld, July 1990, p. 145.

[2] Ibid., p. 145.

[3] Wendy Taylor, "Don't Let Your Monitor Be the Death of You," *PC Computing,* pp. 228-229.

[4] Diana Hembree, "Warning: Computing Can Be Hazardous To Your Health," *MacWorld,* January 1990, pp. 150-157.

[5] Deborah Branscum, Column, Conspicuous Consumer, "Rating Radiation Screens," *MacWorld,* July 1990, p. 84.

[6] Bristol Voss, "Health Hazards: Hidden Perils in the Workplace," *Sales & Marketing Management,* November 1991, pp. 127-128.

[7] Interview, May 3, 1993, with Louis Slesin.

APPENDIX

WHICH EYE DOCTOR
TO GO TO

Picture a visit to the eye doctor.

What do you think of? An eye chart on the wall on one side of the examining room and you sitting in a chair on the opposite side trying to read the tiny letters on the bottom line of the chart across the room. Right?

And, if you *can* read the bottom line, your vision is perfect. If you can't, you need glasses. Right? — Well, not necessarily!

Blurred vision — the tip of the iceberg

Blurred vision is only one of the eye and vision symptoms of Computer Stress Syndrome and is usually preceded by an unnoticed decline in the Critical Visual Skills.

Don't wait until you experience blurred vision before seeing a behavioral optometrist. If you wait until then, you've waited too long and may have lost the opportunity to halt further decline.

It is time to go to a behavioral optometrist when you first notice *any* of the symptoms described in this book. Even better, you should go *before* any symptoms appear. We suggest that you see a behavioral optometrist when you start using a computer and, thereafter, at least once a year.

It's important to remember that poor vision is not inevitable and not irreversible. A behavioral optometrist will often offer a program of vision therapy that enhances vision through exercise, relaxation and training.

Even if you can read the bottom line on the chart there could be other hidden visual deficiencies that might affect your comfort and efficiency at the computer.

Efficient visual performance at the computer requires more than sharp acuity (clarity of vision). In addition to acuity, there are five other visual skills that the eyes perform. These six visual skills are called the Critical Visual Skills.

(For a detailed explanation of the Critical Visual Skills necessary for computer work, see How The Eyes Work At The Computer, Pp. 95 - 98.)

Undetected deficiencies in the Critical Visual Skills are often the underlying cause of eye and vision symptoms of Computer Stress Syndrome.

Only a comprehensive vision exam can determine the level of functioning of your Critical Visual Skills.

The Ideal Visit

Here is a list of the vision checks and tests that a behavioral optometrist performs during the first visit:

- Measure distance vision with an eye chart.
- Determine how your eyes function at close range.
- Measure the teamwork between your eyes and your brain.
- See how smoothly your eyes move from point to point.
- See how smoothly and easily your eyes follow a moving target.
- See how easily each eye can shift focus from near to far.
- Screen for medical conditions like glaucoma and cataracts.

If you are already using glasses, or suffer from any of the eye or vision symptoms of Computer Stress Syndrome, this comprehensive testing can determine the most effective approach to your vision care.

This complete series of tests can also determine whether or not you could benefit from a vision training program.

One the other hand, using glasses that were prescribed after only one test for acuity could very likely lead to further visual stress, prescriptions that get stronger, and a general feeling of discomfort and, perhaps, overall fatigue.

To help the behavioral optometrist determine the "computer glasses" that would be best for you, bring a sketch showing all the distances at which you need to see your work area. This would include the distances to the computer screen, keyboard, the original copy you work from and to any other materials that you use. Measure distance to the screen from the bridge of your nose.

What is behavioral optometry?

A behavioral optometrist has received specialized training in detecting deficiencies in the Critical Visual Skills. In addition, a behavioral optometrist can provide a training program that improves visual functioning. Of course, a behavioral optometrist, like a regular optometrist, can also prescribe glasses and contacts.

A behavioral optometrist is best qualified to decide if "computer glasses" would be appropriate and to prescribe the kind you need. He or she can also provide you with a customized training program that could restore and/or enhance your Critical Visual Skills.

How to find a behavioral optometrist

To locate a behavioral optometrist in your area contact one of these sources:

College of Optometrists in Vision Development
P.O. Box 285
Chula Vista, CA 92012
(619) 425-6191

Optometric Extension Program Foundation
2912 S. Daimler Street
Santa Ana, CA 92705
(714) 250-8070

American Optometric Association
243 N. Lindbergh Blvd.
St. Louis, MO 63141
(314) 991-4100

When you have the name of someone, it is perfectly reasonable to telephone the doctor and ask whether he or she does a complete series of tests described in The Ideal Visit and whether he or she prescribes special "computer glasses." (See Which Glasses To Use At The Computer, Pp. 33 - 34)

It is also useful to inquire whether vision therapy is available in the office. This would indicate that the doctor is behaviorally trained.

A NOTE TO EMPLOYERS

On the one hand, it is the responsibility of each individual to seek out the information and techniques that can make him or her more healthy, effective and productive at the computer.

On the other, many corporations are recognizing that by providing both the proper work environment and the proper training for computer operators they can retain a competitive edge and control health costs.

Proper application of the principles in **Total Health At The Computer** can lead to increased productivity, greater employee comfort, morale and well being and reduced insurance claims.

Consulting and training services available from the Cambridge Institute for Better Vision include:

1. Consulting to designers, business owners and others in optimal office design and set up for computer work areas;
2. In-house training of personnel in the application of the principles of **Total Health At The Computer** and;
3. "Train the trainer" certification programs for consultants, trainers and human resource people.

For more information contact:

Martin Sussman
Cambridge Institute
65 Wenham Road
Topsfield, MA 01983
PH: (508) 887-3883
FAX: (508) 887-3885

The following four eye charts are to be used with some of the exercises of the 3-minute routines and the Vision Enhancement Training.

Each eye chart is printed on its own page so that you can cut them out to use them.

Alternatively, you can order large-size copies of the charts from the Cambridge Institute, 65 Wenham Road, Topsfield MA 01983. Each chart is $1.00.

COMPUTER EYECHART

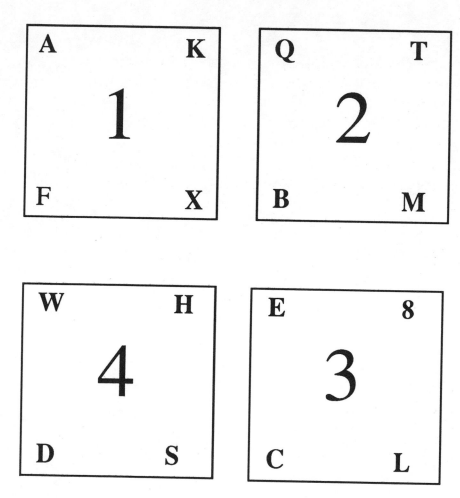

+ CHART

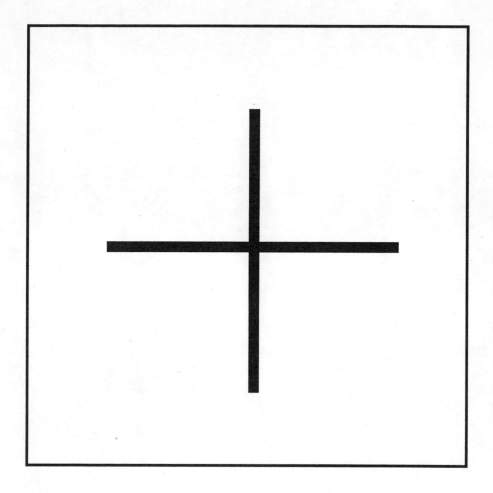

LARGE LETTER CHART

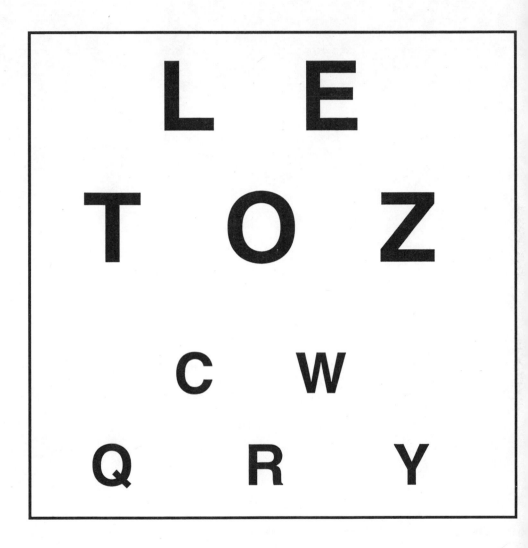

SMALL LETTER CHART

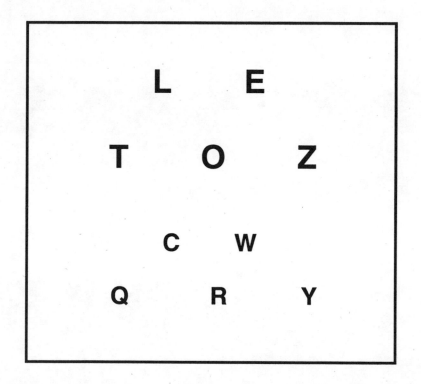

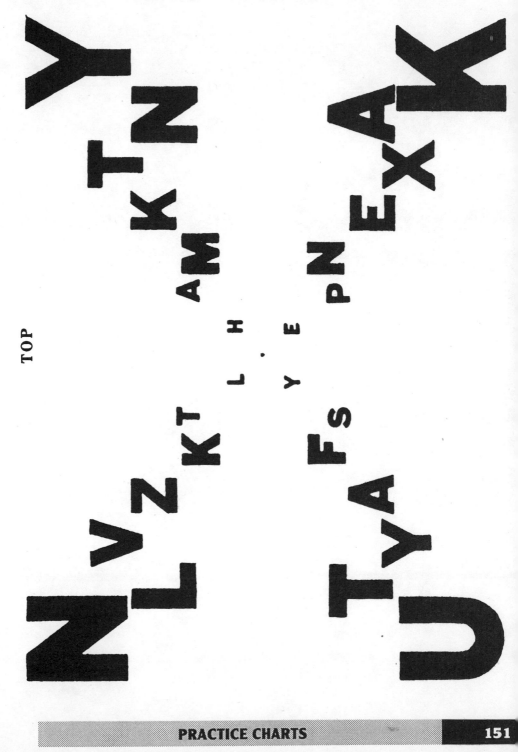

INDEX

ABOUT THE AUTHORS

Martin A. Sussman, founder and Executive Director of the Cambridge Institute for Better Vision in Topsfield, Massachusetts, has been teaching natural vision improvement for 16 years. In 1977, he co-created the EYECLASSES Seminar, a weekend vision training that he still facilitates. He has been publishing *The Program for Better Vision*, a comprehensive, home-study vision-improvement course, since 1985. He conducts weekly classes and one-day workshops, offers private lessons and lectures throughout the United States and Canada. He holds a B.A. in psychology from Rutgers University.

Dr. Ernest V. Loewenstein, Ph.D., O.D., practices optometry in Newton, Massachusetts, and is Associate Professor of Optics at The New England College of Optometry in Boston. In his private practice he places special emphasis on vision training and on vision-related learning problems. He lectures within his field and to educators in teaching professions. In 1989, he was named Optometrist of the Year by the Massachusetts Society of Optometrists. A graduate of The New England College of Optometry, he holds a B.S. in science from Cornell University and a Ph.D. in physics, with a concentration in optics, from Johns Hopkins University.

Howard Sann, a writer and editor based in Bridgeport, Connecticut, seemed sentenced to a lifetime in glasses until he took Mr. Sussman's vision seminar in 1982. A year and a half later, after working with Dr. Carl Gruning, a Fairfield, Conn., behavioral optometrist, he shed the glasses he'd worn since 1950. He restored his vision over an 18-month period during which he was working long hours at the computer, despite less than optimum conditions: glare-ridden VDT screens and poorly lit offices. A contributor to books for more than 20 years, he runs Victory Ink, a publicity and promotion company. He edited *The Program for Better Vision* as well as this book. He is a 1965 graduate of Lafayette College.

ADDITIONAL PRODUCTS AND SERVICES FROM THE CAMBRIDGE INSTITUTE

The Cambridge Institute also provides these products and services:

1. Training materials and full-sized versions of the charts that are used in this book.

2. Audio tape home-study programs for improving vision and maintaining health and relaxation.

3. On-site training and consulting in the principles of **Total Health at the Computer**.

4. Ergonomically designed products that support comfort, relaxation and productivity in the work environment.

If you are interested in more detailed information about any of the above, please contact the:

Cambridge Institute
65 Wenham Road
Topsfield MA 01983
PH: 508-887-3883
FAX: 508-887-3885

Other Books on Health and Healing
from Station Hill Press

Overcoming Migraine
A Comprehensive Guide to Treatment and Prevention by a Survivor
Revised and Expanded Edition
BETSY WYCKOFF

This landmark guide explains and evaluates the full range of chemical, dietary and alternative therapies currently available for migraine headaches. The author, who was once a migraine sufferer, provides a unique perspective on this debilitating disorder, and offers the welcome news that millions are suffering needlessly—migraines can be prevented. She points out how often the reactions are due to allergies, particularly to certain foods; she describes the factors that can trigger an attack, and discusses the range of available treatments and her own responses to them. This revised and enlarged edition contains new chapters dealing with migraine in children and the elderly, anecdotal remedies, and unorthodox approaches to migraine management such as homeopathy and oriental medicine. Also included are letters from readers of the first edition of this book, sharing their treatment experiences.

$10.95 paper, ISBN 0-88268-126-5

Do You Really Need Eyeglasses?
DR. MARILYN B. ROSANES-BERRETT

Growing evidence indicates that the vast majority of eye difficulties are rooted in tension and poor use of eye muscles. The simple exercises presented in this book can help anyone become eye-glass free. The author herself was beset with hyperopia, astigmatism, and crossed eyes, yet today she does not wear glasses. Her revolutionary technique, the first to combine Bates and Gestalt therapy to attain maximum vision, is based on a series of easily performed training procedures designed to improve circulation, relax the muscles of the eyes, avoid strain, and arrest deterioration. This expanded edition includes eye techniques for total relaxation as well as up-to-date information on a range of optical problems including: computer eye strain, poor peripheral vision, night blindness, glaucoma, myopia and astigmatism.

$10.95 paper, ISBN 0-88268-104-4, $20.95 cloth, ISBN 0-88268-107-9.

How to Forgive
When You Don't Know How
JACQUI BISHOP AND MARY GRUNTE

In this groundbreaking look at the psychology of forgiveness, the authors show how resentment toward other people, toward one's self, even toward God can consume precious emotional energy and seriously impair both self-esteem and the ability to experience joy. Drawing on the healing techniques used so successfully in *How to Love Yourself When You Don't Know How*, they offer a short program for accelerating the process of forgiveness, including visualization, emotional discharge, searching back, and prayer. Envlivened with classic quotations on the nature of forgiveness, this revolutionary book explodes long-standing myths including the notion that forgiveness involves self-denial, making up, confessing, or turning the other cheek. Its easy-to-use format puts it on the shelf with *Good Grief Rituals*.

A HEALING COMPANION $8.95 paper, ISBN 0-88268-142-7

How to Love Yourself
When You Don't Know How
Healing All Your Inner Children
JACQUI BISHOP AND MARY GRUNTE

The notion that each of us carries around an inner child has been widely explored in popular psychology; this groundbreaking book takes the premise one step further, describing an interior model for the individual based on the metaphor of the family. Everyone, say the authors, is really made up of an inner family—several children of various ages and characters, each of whom vies for control in one's life, as well as an inner grownup capable of learning to care for them. The book's aim is to help the reader re-educate the inner grownup to love unconditionally, opening the way for profound healing of psychic wounds.

$10.95 paper, ISBN 0-88268131-1

Good Grief Rituals

Tools for Healing

ELAINE CHILDS-GOWELL

As a psychotherapist with over 20 year's experience, the author realized that the emotion of grief was not limited to bereavement but was in fact experienced in an extraordinary range of circumstances, from natural disasters to the end of a love affair. In this sane, comforting, and deeply thoughtful book, she offers the reader a series of simple grief rituals, among them the venting of feelings, letter writing, affirmations, exercises to act out negative emotions as well as forgiveness, fantasies, meditations, and more. Adult children of alcoholics and dysfunctional families, victims of incest and assault, and those who've lost a beloved or a pet, wrecked a car, or suffered any kind of loss, will find that these "good grief rituals" move them through loss to forgiveness and, ultimately, to gratitude and a new sense of life.

A HEALING COMPANION $8.95 paper, ISBN 0-88268-118-4

Emotional First Aid

A Crisis Handbook

SEAN HALDANE, M.D.

Emotional First Aid is the first book to address immediate emotional crisis as distinct from a person's general state of mental health. It deals with grief, anger, fear, joy, and also the complex feelings of parent/child conflicts—emotions that can lead to further withdrawal, illness, or even violence. Clear and extraordinarily well written, this is the first book to draw on Reichian character analysis to explain how differences in individuals and in specific emotions call for different responses, if one is to be supportive and not invasive. Emotional first aid may precede or prevent therapy in the same way that physical first aid can precede or prevent extended medical treatment.

$9.95 paper, ISBN 0-88268-071-4

How To Break the Vicious Circles in Your Relationships

A Guide for Couples

DEE ANNA PARRISH, MSSW

The message of this clear and sympathetic book is that dysfunctional relationships—characterized by a predictable pattern of vicious circles— can be healed. Reassuring case histories drawn from the author's own therapeutic practice demonstrate why relationships disintegrate and show how they can be made whole again. Here are proven techniques designed to short-circuit destructive habits. Readers will learn to use "defusers" to keep conflicts from escalating, gauge levels of emotional intimacy and identify barriers to closeness, examine their own levels of communication and quality of listening, use "I" statements to identify problematic issues, and uncover inter-generational patterns of dysfunction. For anyone seeking to improve a relationship or reconnect with a partner—with or without the aid of a therapist—this is essential reading.

A HEALING COMPANION $8.95 paper, ISBN 0-88268-144-3

Abused

A Guide to Recovery for Adult Survivors of Emotional/Physical Child Abuse

DEE ANNA PARRISH, MSSW

This clear and sensitively written book covers child abuse in all its forms, including types of abuse overlooked by the victims themselves: neglect, deprivation, ridicule, and inappropriate sexual gestures. *Abused* includes a wealth of revealing and highly moving first-person accounts, a program for recovery, a resource directory, and various self-tests to help readers determine if they once were abused and today need counselling or therapy. It includes a parents' guide to behavioral signs of sexual abuse plus the first guide to describe techniques used by therapists to uncover repressed memories. Illustrated with case histories, *Abused* is written for adults who suspect the treatment they received as children still impairs their sense of judgment and well-being today.

$10.95 paper, ISBN 0-88268-089-7

These titles are available from your local bookstore or directly from:
Station Hill Press
Barrytown, New York 12507
Write for a free catalogue